Abdominoplasty

Editors

ALAN MATARASSO
JAMES E. ZINS

CLINICS IN
PLASTIC SURGERY

www.plasticsurgery.theclinics.com

July 2020 • Volume 47 • Number 3

ELSEVIER

1600 John F. Kennedy Boulevard • Suite 1800 • Philadelphia, Pennsylvania, 19103-2899

http://www.theclinics.com

CLINICS IN PLASTIC SURGERY Volume 47, Number 3
July 2020 ISSN 0094-1298, ISBN-13: 978-0-323-75973-1

Editor: Stacy Eastman
Developmental Editor: Nicole Congleton

Clinics in Plastic Surgery (ISSN 0094-1298) is published quarterly by Elsevier Inc., 360 Park Avenue South, New York, NY 10010-1710. Months of issue are January, April, July, and October. Business and Editorial Offices: 1600 John F. Kennedy Blvd., Suite 1800, Philadelphia, PA 19103-2899. Periodicals postage paid at New York, NY and additional mailing offices. Subscription prices are $543.00 per year for US individuals, $987.00 per year for US institutions, $100.00 per year for US students and residents, $607.00 per year for Canadian individuals, $1175.00 per year for Canadian institutions, $655.00 per year for international individuals, $1175.00 per year for international institutions, $100.00 per year for Canadian and $305.00 per year for international students/residents. To receive student/resident rate, orders must be accompanied by name of affiliated institution, date of term, and the *signature* of program/residency coordinator on institution letterhead. Orders will be billed at individual rate until proof of status is received. Foreign air speed delivery is included in all *Clinics* subscription prices. All prices are subject to change without notice. **POSTMASTER:** Send address changes to *Clinics in Plastic Surgery*, Elsevier Health Sciences Division, Subscription Customer Service, 3251 Riverport Lane, Maryland Heights, MO 63043. **Customer Service: 1-800-654-2452 (US and Canada). From outside of the United States and Canada, call 314-447-8871. Fax: 314-447-8029. E-mail: JournalsCustomerService-usa@elsevier.com (for print support); JournalsOnlineSupport-usa@elsevier.com (for online support).**

Reprints. For copies of 100 or more of articles in this publication, please contact the Commercial Reprints Department, Elsevier Inc., 360 Park Avenue South, New York, New York 10010-1710. Tel.: +1-212-633-3874; Fax: +1-212-633-3820; E-mail: reprints@elsevier.com.

Clinics in Plastic Surgery is covered in *Current Contents, EMBASE/Excerpta Medica, Science Citation Index, MEDLINE/PubMed (Index Medicus), ASCA, and ISI/BIOMED.*

Contributors

EDITORS

ALAN MATARASSO, MD, FACS
Clinical Professor of Surgery, Donald and
Barbara Zucker School of Medicine at Hofstra/
Northwell, New York, New York, USA

JAMES E. ZINS, MD, FACS
Chair, Department of Plastic Surgery,
Cleveland Clinic, Program Director, Cleveland
Clinic Post Graduate Aesthetic Fellowship,
Professor of Surgery, Cleveland Clinic Lerner
College of Medicine, Cleveland, Ohio, USA

AUTHORS

AMY K. ALDERMAN, MD, MPH
North Atlanta Plastic Surgery, Alpharetta,
Georgia, USA

CARLOS ALTAMIRANO-ARCOS, MD
Hospital General "Dr. Manuel Gea González,"
Mexico City, Mexico

JONATHAN P. BROWER, MD
Body Contouring Fellow, Department of
Plastic Surgery, University of Pittsburgh
Medical Center, Pittsburgh, Pennsylvania,
USA

LUCIANO NAHAS COMBINA, MD
Hospital General "Dr. Manuel Gea González,"
Mexico City, Mexico

CLAIRE E.E. DE VRIES, MD
Department of Surgery, Brigham and Women's
Hospital, Boston, Massachusetts, USA

CARLOS GOYENECHE, MD
Serviço de Cirurgia Plástica Osvaldo Saldanha,
Clinica Saldanha, Departament of Plastic
Surgery, Universidade Metropolitana de
Santos, Santos, Sao Paulo, Brazil

MAARTEN M. HOOGBERGEN, MD, PhD
Department of Plastic and Reconstructive
Surgery, Catharina Hospital, Eindhoven, The
Netherlands

ALFREDO E. HOYOS ARIZA, MD
Plastic and Cosmetic Surgeon, Member of the
International Society of Aesthetic Plastic
Surgery (ISAPS), Member of the Colombian
Society of Aesthetic and Reconstructive
Plastic Surgery (SCCP), Private Practice,
Bogota, Colombia

DENNIS J. HURWITZ, MD
Clinical Professor of Plastic Surgery, Director,
Hurwitz Center for Plastic Surgery, Pittsburgh,
Pennsylvania, USA

JEFFREY E. JANIS, MD, FACS
Professor of Plastic Surgery, Neurosurgery,
Neurology, and Surgery, Department of
Plastic Surgery, The Ohio State University
Wexner Medical Center, Columbus, Ohio,
USA

ANNE F. KLASSEN, DPhil
McMaster University, Hamilton, Ontario,
Canada

CASEY T. KRAFT, MD
Resident, Department of Plastic Surgery, The
Ohio State University Wexner Medical Center,
Columbus, Ohio, USA

ANDRÉS I. ORDENES, MD
Serviço de Cirurgia Plástica Osvaldo Saldanha,
Clinica Saldanha, Departament of Plastic

Surgery, Universidade Metropolitana de Santos, Santos, Sao Paulo, Brazil

NICOLAS OYARCE, MD
Serviço de Cirurgia Plástica Osvaldo Saldanha, Clinica Saldanha, Departament of Plastic Surgery, Universidade Metropolitana de Santos, Santos, Sao Paulo, Brazil

MAURICIO E. PEREZ PACHON, MD
Medical Doctor, Editor and researcher, Private Practice, Bogota, Colombia

MARTHA PAREDES, MD
Serviço de Cirurgia Plástica Osvaldo Saldanha, Clinica Saldanha, Departament of Plastic Surgery, Universidade Metropolitana de Santos, Santos, Sao Paulo, Brazil

HARLAN POLLOCK, MD, FACS
Private Practice, Retired, Clinical Instructor, University of Texas Southwestern, Dallas, Texas, USA

TODD A. POLLOCK, MD, FACS
Private Practice, Clinical Associate Professor, University of Texas Southwestern, Dallas, Texas, USA

ANDREA L. PUSIC, MD, MSc
Department of Surgery, Brigham and Women's Hospital, Boston, Massachusetts, USA

J. PETER RUBIN, MD, FACS
Chairperson, Department of Plastic Surgery, University of Pittsburgh

Medical Center, Pittsburgh, Pennsylvania, USA

AHMAD SAAD, MD, FACS
IMAGN Institute, Barcelona, Spain

CRISTIANNA BONETTO SALDANHA, MD
Serviço de Cirurgia Plástica Osvaldo Saldanha, Clinica Saldanha, Departament of Plastic Surgery, Universidade Metropolitana de Santos, Santos, Sao Paulo, Brazil

OSVALDO SALDANHA, MD, PhD
Serviço de Cirurgia Plástica Osvaldo Saldanha, Clinica Saldanha, Director, Departament of Plastic Surgery, Universidade Metropolitana de Santos, Santos, Sao Paulo, Brazil

OSVALDO SALDANHA FILHO, MD
Serviço de Cirurgia Plástica Osvaldo Saldanha, Clinica Saldanha, Departament of Plastic Surgery, Universidade Metropolitana de Santos, Santos, Sao Paulo, Brazil

MICHELE A. SHERMAK, MD
Associate Professor of Plastic Surgery, Johns Hopkins Department of Plastic Surgery, Private Practice, Plastic Surgeon, Lutherville, Maryland, USA

LAUREN WRIGHT, DO
Fellow, Hurwitz Center for Plastic Surgery, Pittsburgh, Pennsylvania, USA

Contents

> Lipoabdominoplasty is one of the most frequent abdominal body contouring pro-
> cedures performed today. It guarantees a safe combination of abdominoplasty and
> liposuction while minimizing the risk of ischemic flap complications. This is
> because of the limited undermining performed and the liposuction adjunct, both
> of which minimize perforator injury. In the last several years, the integration of
> anatomic definition through the use of liposuction has further refined the proced-
> ure, led to improved results, and increased patient satisfaction. The more natural
> results of the anatomic abdominal definition is a next step in abdominal contour
> refinement.

> Drain-free abdominoplasty using progressive tension sutures (PTS) was initially
> described in 2000 in a small retrospective series. However, the authors' experi-
> ence with this technique spans well over 3 decades, and their technique has
> evolved to simplify the procedure to make it easier and more reproducible by
> the surgeon and improve the patient's recovery and overall experience. This
> article provides in-depth technical details on the authors' no-drain abdomino-
> plasty technique. The authors also address through recent literature some of
> the commonly stated barriers to surgeons instituting this technique into their ab-
> dominoplasty procedure, including excessive time of placement, dimpling, and
> effectiveness.

 Video content accompanies this article at http://www.plasticsurgery.theclinics.com.

> Abdominoplasty is the fifth most common cosmetic plastic surgery procedure
> performed in the United States and combining it with other procedures has
> become more the norm than the outlier. Liposuction is the most common adjunc-
> tive procedure, followed by breast surgery, lower back lift, and thigh lift, in addi-
> tion to hernia repair and gynecologic procedures. The goal of these combination
> procedures includes creating more global aesthetic improvement while protecting
> patients from complications, based on consideration of confounding medical vari-
> ables and increased risks presented by surgery of prolonged duration and
> exposure.

Noninvasive and minimally invasive treatments are increasingly supplanting, or complimenting, abdominoplasty. For optimal delivery of patient care and to maintain a dominant share of the body-contouring market, plastic surgeons need to embrace these new technologies. High capital purchases, costly disposables, maintenance fees, lack of experience, conflicting anecdotal reports, energy-related complications, marketing hyperbole, and rapid obsolescence are formidable barriers to this adoption. Receptive plastic surgeons may be best served by accepting brief short-term retrospective reports by reputable innovative body contouring surgeons who present a succinct and clinically supported message.

After massive weight loss (MWL), patients present with deformities that are more severe and often different than those observed in standard cosmetic abdominoplasty. The first step is careful consideration of the special factors involved in preoperative screening of patients with MWL presenting for body contouring surgery. Once these patient factors are optimized and surgery is considered, careful analysis of anatomic deformities should ensue. Technical variations of standard abdominoplasty are often required. With proper attention to safe screening, analysis of the anatomic deformities, and application of relevant techniques, plastic surgeons can have a positive impact on the lives of these patients.

Abdominal etching techniques are used to improve the aesthetics of the abdominal region, providing patients an athletic physique, using liposuction and fat redistribution. Based on the anatomy of fat layers, lipocontouring for deep fat liposuction and superficial fat liposculpting for superficial fat liposuction are proposed. The degree of abdominal etching is controlled by the surgeon through the extent of lipocontouring and superficial fat liposculpting. Therefore, we propose the classification of low-, medium-, and high-definition abdominal etching levels. This article offers a comprehensive description of the authors' technique, including preoperative assessment, intraoperative procedure, and postoperative care for patients undergoing abdominal etching.

Abdominoplasty is a commonly performed aesthetic procedure but has one of the highest risks for venous thromboembolism (VTE) events in aesthetic surgery. Surgeons can face challenging decisions when performing combination procedures and deciding on appropriate methods of VTE prophylaxis. This article summarizes the current evidence for the incidence of VTE events in abdominoplasty and abdominoplasty combined with other procedures, the current recommendations for risk stratification and management, and options available for mechanical and chemical VTE prophylaxis.

High-Definition Excisional Body Contouring: Mini Lipoabdominoplasty (FIT Mommy) and Enhanced Viability Abdominoplasty

Alfredo E. Hoyos Ariza and Mauricio E. Perez Pachon

The abdominoplasty procedure poses a number of unique challenges. If the stigmata of the operation is to be avoided, careful planning and surgical execution are required. We describe our experience in full and mini abdominoplasties with a 360-degree approach, involving all muscular groups and body segments as described by high-definition liposculpture. Selective fat grafting is also safely performed in specific areas to improve projection and volume.

Measuring Outcomes in Cosmetic Abdominoplasty: The BODY-Q

Claire E.E. de Vries, Anne F. Klassen, Maarten M. Hoogbergen, Amy K. Alderman, and Andrea L. Pusic

The BODY-Q is a condition-specific patient-reported outcome measure that enables a comprehensive assessment of outcomes that are specific to patients undergoing body contouring procedures such as abdominoplasty. The BODY-Q scales were designed to be responsive to the effects of abdominoplasty on health-related quality of life and appearance outcomes. The BODY-Q covers a range of content domains, and the independently functioning scales enable surgeons to tailor the BODY-Q to their needs. The application of the BODY-Q in cosmetic clinics internationally may give rise to better understanding of abdominoplasty outcomes and optimize the care delivered to patients undergoing these procedures.

CLINICS IN PLASTIC SURGERY

ISSUE OF RELATED INTEREST

Facial Plastic Surgery Clinics
https://www.facialplastic.theclinics.com/
Otolaryngologic Clinics
https://www.oto.theclinics.com/

THE CLINICS ARE AVAILABLE ONLINE!
Access your subscription at:
www.theclinics.com

Preface
Abdominoplasty: State-of-the-Art

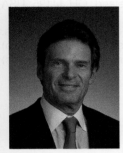   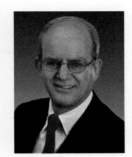

Alan Matarasso, MD, FACS   James E. Zins, MD, FACS

Editors

While journal articles are instructive, they may often give the reader a single surgeon's perspective. Furthermore, the article may or may not compare and contrast the author's results with the previous plastic surgery literature. Continuing Medical Education (CME) articles may address a topic of clinical importance in its entirety but often lack sufficient detail due to journal space constraints.

This *Clinics in Plastic Surgery* issue is different. The purpose of this issue is to cover a range of treatment options and describe them in sufficient detail to allow the practicing plastic surgeon to incorporate the given procedure seamlessly into his or her practice.

Aesthetic improvement in the appearance of the abdomen has always been a priority of patients and indeed is often the cornerstone of the body-contouring procedure. Statistics compiled regarding surgery and nonsurgical treatments attest to the public's unabated concerns. This issue of 9 articles is designed to address the current state-of-the-art in abdominoplasty surgery and related abdominal contouring options. Plastic surgery has evolved from the traditional dermolipectomy with sheet–to-sheet dissection and the associated harmful effects to blood supply and the ensuing high complication rate, to a more nuanced approach: reduced extent of flap dissection based on blood supply anatomy, the option of quilting sutures, the inclusion of ancillary procedures when indicated, and even the introduction of new minimally invasive technologies.

The strength of the multiauthored publication is in the quality of the contributors. We are fortunate that all of our first-choice authors accepted our invitation and provided articles in a timely manner. Each article is written by an authority who details his or her technique in exquisite detail. The discussions compare and contrast the authors' surgical results with the previous literature. The articles are well illustrated, and the results are uniformly outstanding.

The issue is appropriate for both the less experienced and the most experienced plastic surgeons. Both will take important lessons away from the reading.

When read cover to cover, this issue addresses the gamut of important aspects of this topic, and the reader will have acquired an in-depth understanding of the current state of abdominal body-contouring surgery.

Alan Matarasso, MD, FACS
Hofstra University/
Northwell School of Medicine
1009 Park Avenue
New York, NY 10028, USA

Clin Plastic Surg 47 (2020) ix–x
https://doi.org/10.1016/j.cps.2020.03.009
0094-1298/20/© 2020 Published by Elsevier Inc.

James E. Zins, MD, FACS
Department of Plastic Surgery
Cleveland Clinic
Cleveland Clinic Lerner College
of Medicine
9500 Euclid Avenue, A60
Cleveland, OH 44195, USA

E-mail addresses:
amatarasso@drmatarasso.com (A. Matarasso)
zinsj@ccf.org (J.E. Zins)

Lipoabdominoplasty with Anatomic Definition
An Evolution on Saldanha's Technique

Osvaldo Saldanha, MD, PhD*, Andrés I. Ordenes, MD,
Carlos Goyeneche, MD, Nicolas Oyarce, MD, Martha Paredes, MD,
Osvaldo Saldanha Filho, MD, Cristianna Bonetto Saldanha, MD

KEYWORDS

• Lipoabdominoplasty • Body contouring • Abdominoplasty • Lipectomy • Panniculectomy

KEY POINTS

• Lipoabdominoplasty preserves abdominal wall vascular anatomy through the preservation of the perforating vessels. Dead space is also reduced.
• Liposuction-initiated anatomic definition using individualized marking increases abdominal contour and aesthetic results.
• Perforator preservation and Scarpa fascia suspension are the fundamental reasons for the decreased morbidity with this technique.
• It is a standardized step-by-step technique that is safe and easily reproducible by the practicing plastic surgeon. It will result in optimal aesthetic results when incorporated into one's practice.
• Because patients worldwide are demanding liposuction combined procedures, surgeons should be familiar with this technique.

INTRODUCTION

The aesthetic and functional deformities of the abdomen are characterized by skin flaccidity, lipodystrophy, and diastasis of the rectus abdominis muscles.

In the last two decades, lipoabdominoplasty (LAP) has changed the concepts regarding abdominal flap undermining. Limited undermining combined with liposuction has replaced the wide undermining of the traditional abdominoplasty. The result is a preservation of the important abdominal perforators of the deep inferior epigastric artery and a significant reduction in ischemic flap problems postoperatively.[1–5] In addition the patient notes a better aesthetic result and improvement in body contour.

Although the technique is reproducible and aesthetically satisfactory for most patients when performed step by step according to our described technique,[5] one adverse sequelae is an overly flat lower abdomen.

The anatomic abdominal muscular definition, or high-definition,[6–8] abdominoplasty came about through retrospective review of our earlier surgical results. Midline definition has ushered in yet a newer phase of abdominal contouring.

PRINCIPLES OF LIPOABDOMINOPLASTY WITH DEFINITION

The fundamental principle of this technique is still the preservation of abdominal wall perforators at the level of the rectus abdominal muscles through careful central undermining (**Fig. 1**) combined with selective liposuction. Individualized marking is

Serviço de Cirurgia Plástica Osvaldo Saldanha, Universidade Metropolitana de Santos, Av. Ana Costa, 146, Cjs 1201-04, Santos, Sao Paulo 11060-000, Brazil
* Corresponding author. Serviço de Cirurgia Plástica Osvaldo Saldanha, Clinica Saldanha, Av. Ana Costa, 146, Cjs 1201-04, Santos, Sao Paulo 11060-000, Brazil.
E-mail address: clinicasaldanha@hotmail.com

Clin Plastic Surg 47 (2020) 335–349
https://doi.org/10.1016/j.cps.2020.03.004

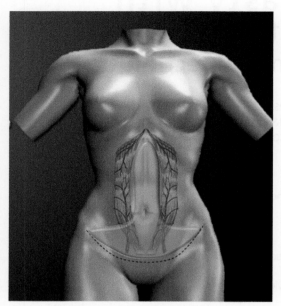

Fig. 1. Surgical undermining. Lipoabdominoplasty preserves vascular perforators from the rectus muscles but allows for an avascular midline tunnel to perform rectus plication. The *dotted line* indicates the incision.

done preoperatively according to the patient's individual anatomy. Some areas will have deep liposuction, others superficial and deep, depending on the proximity of the perforators and the areas to be defined. The preservation of Scarpa fascia brings important benefits to the procedure.

SURGICAL TECHNIQUE
Patient Selection

Ideal patients for the procedure have body mass index (BMI) less than 30, presenting lipodystrophy with abdominal skin laxity. Special attention is given to postbariatric patients (poor skin retraction capability); patients who smoke; and patients who have undergone previous abdominal surgery, including previous abdominal liposuction. Abdominal hernias scars are searched for and noted. These patients may be more amenable for more traditional LAP without definition.

When anatomic definition is done it is important to understand that not every patient will get a high-definition procedure. Most will get a moderate- or even low-definition procedure, depending on BMI, skin quality, and abdominal wall musculature. Because of the variability in patient body type a specific end point in liposuction is hard to define and an artistic point of view combined with an eye on safety is needed. In general, BMI greater than 27 and poor skin quality mitigates against significant definition. Instead, just the creation of a

soft negative concavity, especially in the central area, avoids an artificial appearance and results in a better accommodation of the undermined skin flap.

Marking of the Abdominal Flap and Liposuction Areas

Marking is done preoperatively by drawing a 12- or 14-cm horizontal suprapubic line depending on patient pubic area width that is 5 to 7 cm from the vulvar commissure. Two oblique lines of 7 to 8 cm each are drawn in the direction of the iliac crest within the bikini line completing the inferior incision line; this distance may be longer depending on patient BMI and degree of skin laxity. Next, the supraumbilical limit of the abdominal flap to be resected is marked joining it with the lateral limit of the inferior line (**Fig. 2**).

With the patient lying down rectus anatomy is delineated. The patient is asked to contract the abdominal musculature and the medial and lateral borders of the rectus abdominis muscle are marked as a red area (**Fig. 3**). Thus the diastasis is delineated. The costal margin is also marked.

Three lines are designed for a deep and superficial liposuction (dark green lines): the medial line in the supraumbilical abdomen (linea alba), an inverted subcostal triangle as an abdominal line at the junction of lateral borders of the rectus, with the external oblique muscles (semilunaris lines) (**Fig. 4**). It is important to confirm these lines with the patient in the standing position and with gentle traction of the abdominal flap.

The location of the new umbilicus is marked approximately four fingers above the original umbilicus corresponding to 8 to 10 cm above the pubis (point A, **Figs. 3**B and **4**A). The area below (yellow area) is a reference line used to avoid overly aggressive liposuction because this will be the infraumbilical region of the abdominal flap (see **Fig. 4**).

Finally, the demarcation of the pubic area, flanks, iliac crest, or dorsal region if necessary (light green areas) is performed.

Infiltration

Super wet technique is used, infiltrating all the abdominal region with saline solution and adrenaline (1:500,000), between 1 and 2 L in the abdominal area, prioritizing the areas where more intense liposuction will be performed. The incorporation of an infiltration pump and cannulas can significantly diminish the infiltration time (**Fig. 5**).

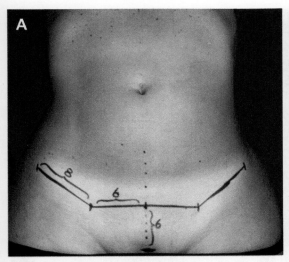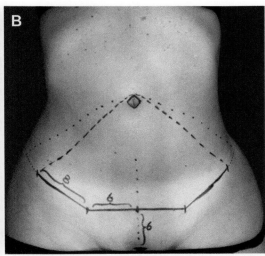

Fig. 2. Personalized abdominal markings. (*A*) Inferior incision design (12-cm horizontal suprapubic line) at 6 cm from the vulvar commissure. Two oblique lines of 8 cm each are drawn in the direction of the iliac crest within the bikini line; *dotted lines* show an extended marking if excessive skin flaccidity exists. (*B*) Supraumbilical limit of the abdominal flap to be resected is marked and joined to the inferior lateral limit of the incision.

Liposuction

Liposuction starts with the patient in the lateral decubitus if dorsal liposuction is performed. The patient is then turned to the opposite lateral decubitus position. First liposuction is made in the dark green areas (areas to be defined), starting in the central region or the linea alba (between the medial edges of the rectus abdominis muscles) and over the position of the new umbilical pedicle (point A, see **Figs. 3**B and 4A). This is done using

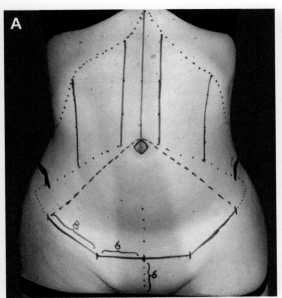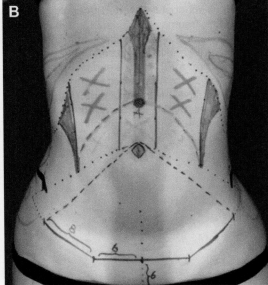

Fig. 3. Individualized markings in dorsal decubitus. (*A*) Possible resection areas of abdominal skin, costal margin, medial and lateral rectal muscle margin, iliac crest limit, and rhomboidal design of umbilicus (*black lines*). (*B*) Possible neoumbilicoplasty position (point A). *Red area*, controlled deep liposuction over rectus abdominal muscles (preservation of perforators). *Yellow area*, moderate and deep liposuction (flap perfusion risk area). *Light green areas*, safe area for intense deep liposuction. *Dark green areas*, area to be defined with superficial and deep liposuction (the semilunaris lines and alba line).

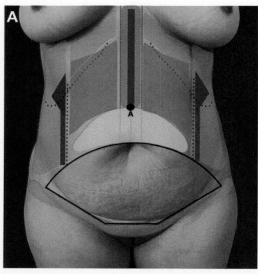
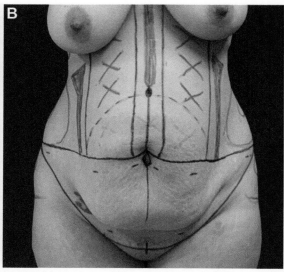

Fig. 4. Individualized markings in standing position. (*A*) Schematic representation of markings. (*B*) Real patient markings. *Black/purple lines*, possible resection areas of abdominal skin, medial and lateral rectal muscle margin, rhomboidal design of umbilicus, incisions for liposuction on the abdominal skin to be resected, and possible neo-umbilicoplasty position (point A). *Red area*, over rectus abdominal muscles (perforators area), note that over the costal margin more liposuction can be performed, that is why in the schematic it is marked as *light green*. *Yellow area*, flap perfusion risk area. *Light green areas*, safe area for intense deep liposuction. *Dark green areas*, area to be defined (alba line and semilunaris lines), note that the subcostal triangle is marked 2 cm over the costal margin because it descends with flap transposition.

conventional cannulas of 3 and 4 mm removing fat first from the superficial layer and then from the deep layer. This is repeated in the semilunaris lines and in the subcostal inverted triangle shape, avoiding the trauma of the subdermal plexus. This is done using cannulas with blunt holes facing down or laterally and leaving a soft transition to the surrounding areas (**Fig. 6**). The end point is to get a pinch test close to 1.5 cm depending on patient BMI, skin quality, and musculature (**Fig. 7**). The horizontal lines of the rectus abdominis or any other horizontal line are not defined, because when the flap is pulled inferiorly these lines may

not be exactly in the anatomic area of the muscle, which may compromise the vascularization of the flap.

Liposuction in the light green areas (flanks, and any posterior areas) is performed in the deep and sometimes superficial layers until achieving a more natural and harmonious outline of the abdominal wall. The pinch test should be between 1.5 and 2 cm (see **Fig. 7**). This new concept of selective liposuction aims to define the natural curves of the abdomen, accentuating areas of muscular insertions. This concept has previously been described by Hoyos.[5–8] Unlike Hoyos we perform selective liposuction, not as aggressive

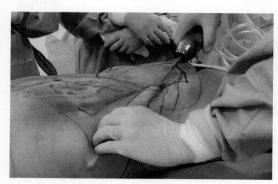

Fig. 5. Infiltration with infiltration pump.

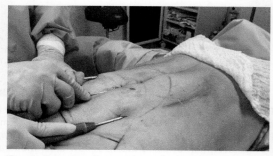

Fig. 6. Selective liposuction of the abdomen with anatomic definition. Liposuction of negative areas.

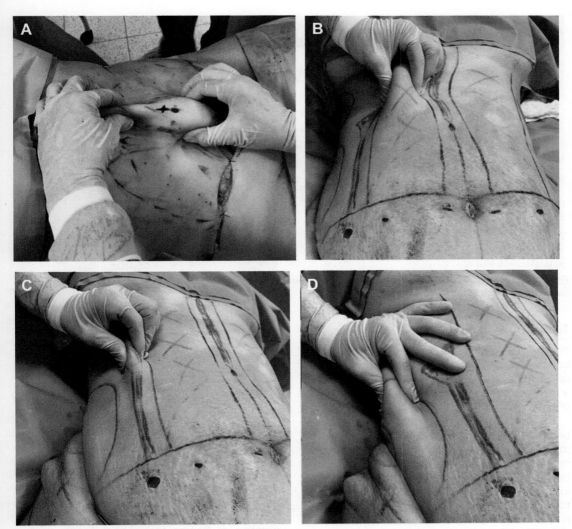

Fig. 7. Pinch test of different areas. (*A*) Definition of alba line (*dark green area*) versus *yellow area* of the flap. (*B*) Perforators area (*red area*). (*C*) Definition of semilunar line (*dark green area*). (*D*) Flank area (*light green area*).

as in the high-definition technique. Instead we aim to establish a natural contour and curves of the abdomen, avoiding the stigma of muscular hypertrophy. We also avoid the use of ultrasound-assisted liposuction. It is our preference to use traditional liposuction, although recently we have begun to use power-assisted liposuction.

Next, liposuction of the red area is done in a deep and controlled way, trying not to injure any perforators of the rectus abdominis. Deep liposuction is done in the yellow area. The pinch test should be between 2.5 and 3 cm, superficial, and some deep fat is also maintained because at the time of resecting the abdominal flap the remaining fat in this area can be resected directly, avoiding excessive trauma to this distal flap region (see **Fig. 7**).

Scarpa Fascia Preservation

The incision of the abdominal skin is done until it reaches the Scarpa fascia, and then the undermining is performed in the suprafascial plane until the level of the anterosuperior iliac spines. This modification on the amount of Scarpa fascia left behind (previously left to the level of umbilicus) was based on the studies and theories of lymphatic preservation, pubic suspension, scar shortening, dead space coaptation, and seroma prevention mentioned in the literature, without creating an inferior abdominal bulge.[9–18] The dissection then continues in the plane of the muscular aponeuroses to the level of umbilicus, under which no liposuction is performed (**Fig. 8**).

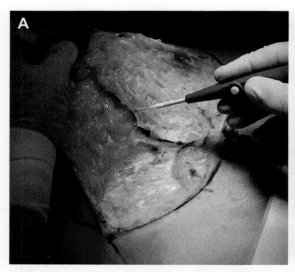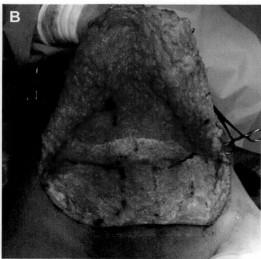

Fig. 8. (*A*) Scarpa fascia preservation until anterior superior iliac spine. (*B*) Central portion of Scarpa fascia overlying the diastasis is removed for complete plication.

Tunnel Undermining

When the infraumbilical undermining its completed, the flap is cut in the middle and the umbilicus is released from the abdominal flap in a rhomboid design and preserved with its pedicle (**Fig. 9**).

The undermining is then continued in the supraumbilical region, between the internal borders of the rectus abdominis muscles avoiding the undermining beyond the middle third of these muscles, because from there some perforators can be injured (**Fig. 10**). Tunnel undermining may reach the xiphoid appendix, depending on the need for rectus muscle plication. The tunnel width may vary with the distance of diastasis because the

perforating vessels follow the muscle separation. To facilitate the muscle plication and to have a better view of the anatomic structures, the Saldanha retractor is used. This is the most important part of LAP, because the preservation of abdominal wall vasculature is the fundamental principle of the technique and its low rate of complication.[19–45]

Plication

In the infraumbilical area, the central portion of Scarpa fascia overlying the diastasis is removed for complete plication of the rectus abdominis from xiphoid appendix to the pubis followed by plication of Scarpa fascia back to the midline and fixed to the rectus abdominis aponeurosis,

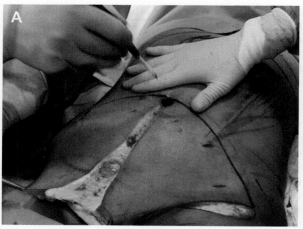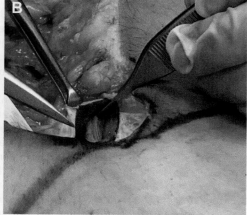

Fig. 9. (*A*) The infraumbilical abdominal is flap cut in the middle. (*B*) Rhomboid umbilical release with its pedicle.

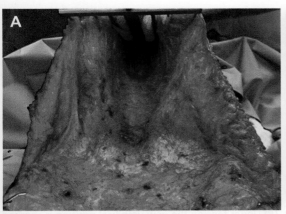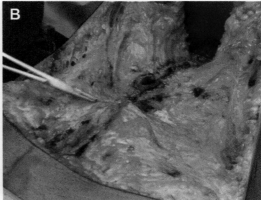

Fig. 10. (*A*) Complete undermining of the tunnel. (*B*) Muscle aponeurosis plication in the midline and Scarpa fascia preservation and suspension.

which creates a great pubic suspension and shortening of the abdominal scar (see **Fig. 10**).

Removing the Infraumbilical Skin Excess

Excess skin of the lower abdomen should be removed after the surgeon makes sure that the flap easily transposes to the pubic symphysis. Liposuction facilitates flap mobilization and blunt cannulas are used to create additional blunt dissection of the flap. In cases where excessive tension is noted in the suture line, sometimes additional lateral dissection is needed to correctly compensate and resolve lateral skin excess, along with dog ear resections.

With the patient sitting in 30° to 40°, the excess skin of the abdominal flap is marked and resected. Also in this step the excess subfascial fat of the lower third of the flap (yellow area) is resected (**Fig. 11**).

Omphaloplasty

After corroboration that the abdominal flap can transpose, the new position of the umbilicus is marked approximately four to five fingers above the final scar and generally over the level of the superior border of the iliac crest (**Fig. 12**), which usually corresponds to the previous demarcation. A star-shaped omphaloplasty is used with a deep fixation of the pedicle (**Fig. 13**).

Suture, Drain, Dressings, and Postoperative Care

The abdomen is sutured in two planes with Monocryl 4–0, in a deep layer (connective/fascial tissue) and another 4–0 layer on the subdermis. At the end of the procedure if there is not much tension on the flap, it is possible to remove about 2 to 3 cm of the pubic skin, placing the scar in a lower position. It is important that the defined semilunar

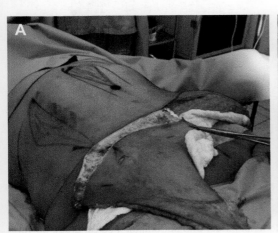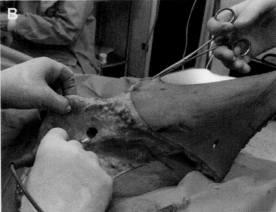

Fig. 11. (*A*) Skin excess resection. (*B*) Direct subfascial fat resection in the yellow area of the flap.

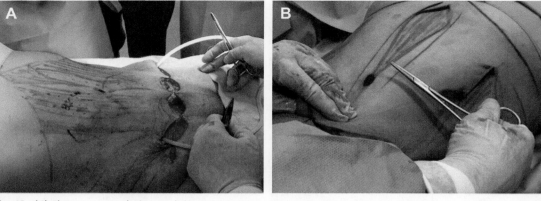

Fig. 12. (*A*) Flap accommodation and drain positioning. (*B*) Under tension the new umbilical position is checked and marked.

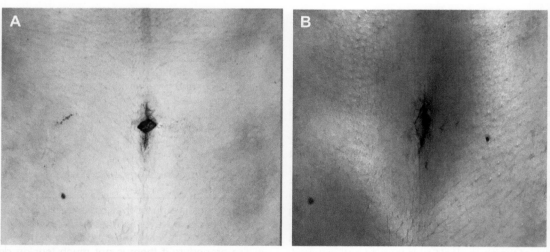

Fig. 13. (*A*) Star-shaped umbilicoplasty. (*B*) Final result.

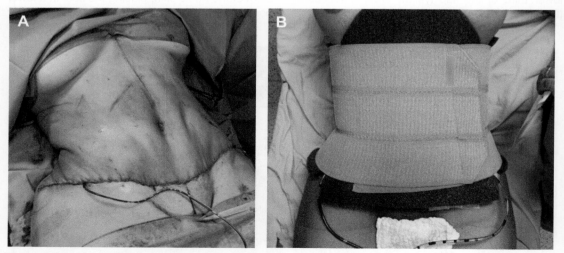

Fig. 14. (*A*) Final result with anatomic definition. (*B*) Abdominal binder and abdominal medical-grade polyurethane foam pads.

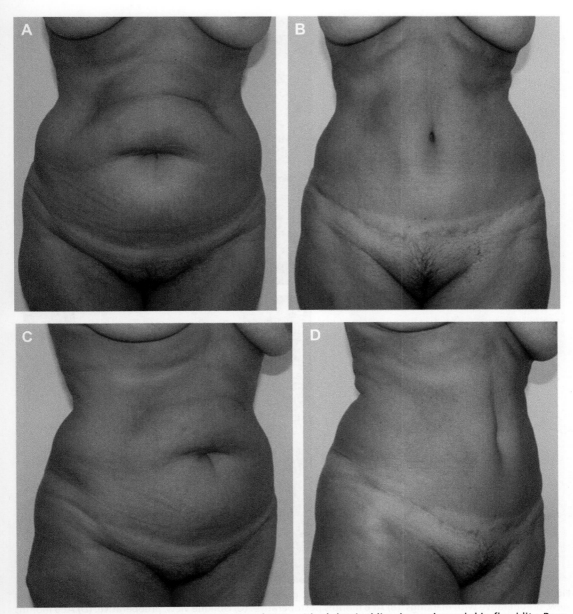

Fig. 15. Clinical case. A 57-year-old patient, BMI of 25.5, with abdominal lipodystrophy and skin flaccidity. Poor skin quality and poor muscular development. (*A*) Frontal view, preoperative. (*B*) At 12 months postoperative. (*C*) Oblique view, preoperative. (*D*) At 12 months postoperative.

lines be sutured symmetrically and toward the pubic tubercle on each side. A continuous aspiration drain is used (**Fig. 14**), which is generally removed when less than 50 mL of fluid is collected in 24 hours, which generally happens on the first postoperative day when the patient is discharged. The dressing is made with Micropore (3M, USA) right in the suture line.

Elastic stocking and intermittent pneumatic compression boot is used until the patient can perform active mobilization. Soft or half-compression garments (abdominal binder or girdles depending on liposuction areas) and abdominal medical-grade polyurethane foam pads, such as Epi-foam (Biodermis, USA), is used for a period of 20 to 30 days (see **Fig. 14**). These compression garments should be checked at the end of surgery

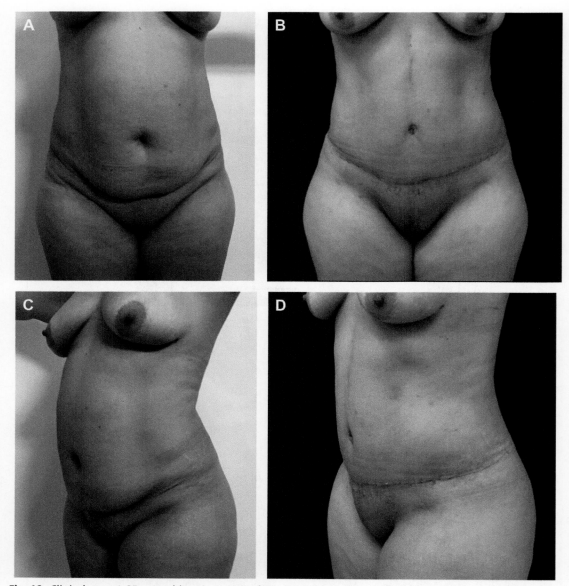

Fig. 16. Clinical case. A 35-year-old patient, BMI of 26, good skin quality and muscular development. (*A*) Frontal view, preoperative with markings. (*B*) At 6 months postoperative. (*C*) Oblique view, preoperative. (*D*) At 6 months postoperative.

to avoid excessive compression on the abdominal flap.

Low-molecular-weight heparin is routinely used postoperatively and continued ambulatory if the patient has risk factors for thromboembolic events for 5 to 7 days. Ambulatory antibiotic prophylaxis is prescribed with first-generation cephalosporin and maintained 24 hours after the drain has been removed. Nonsteroidal anti-inflammatory drugs are prescribed for 5 days, celecoxib (200 mg by

day or divided twice per day if needed) and acetaminophen with codeine (500/30 mg divided every 8 hours only if needed).

In addition, patients benefit from lymphatic drainage, beginning on postoperative day 7.

RESULTS

LAP with anatomic definition is an evolution on the traditional LAP technique. The author has

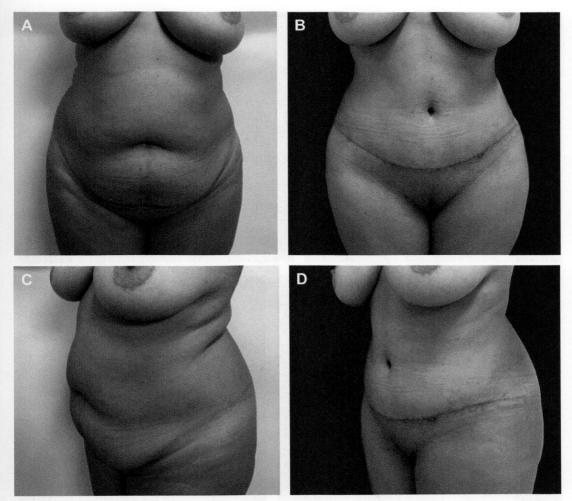

Fig. 17. Clinical case. A 36-year-old patient, BMI of 29, good skin quality, and moderate muscular development. (*A*) Frontal view, preoperative. (*B*) At 8 months postoperative. (*C*) Oblique view, preoperative. (*D*) At 8 months postoperative.

been performing this technique for the last 3 years (starting at 2016). It is the author's opinion and patients' perception that the obtained aesthetic results are superior to the traditional technique because it enhances a natural contour and harmony of the abdomen following the anatomic boundaries of the abdominal wall with maintenance of the safety of traditional LAP (**Figs. 15–18**).

Complication rates have been low: seroma (0%–8%), small skin epitheliolysis less than 1 cm (1%–5%), and hematoma (1%). No cases of skin necrosis or major complications, such as deep vein thrombosis, have been observed. As the definition in general is moderated, no complains about irregularities or need for secondary revision liposuction have happened.

DISCUSSION

Liposuction techniques have changed over time, and that evolution has acquired a high refinement approach to obtain better aesthetics results, but the safety principles when associated with abdominoplasty must be maintained to prevent an increased rate of complications that almost prohibited their combination.[3,4] The abdominal wall vascular territories must be known.[19–25] The superior territory of the abdominal wall in LAP depends on the perforators of the deep epigastric vessels; if they are preserved, aggressive liposuction of the flap is made with low complication rates.[26,27]

Different studies have compared the complication rates in W-pattern abdominoplasty (Heller

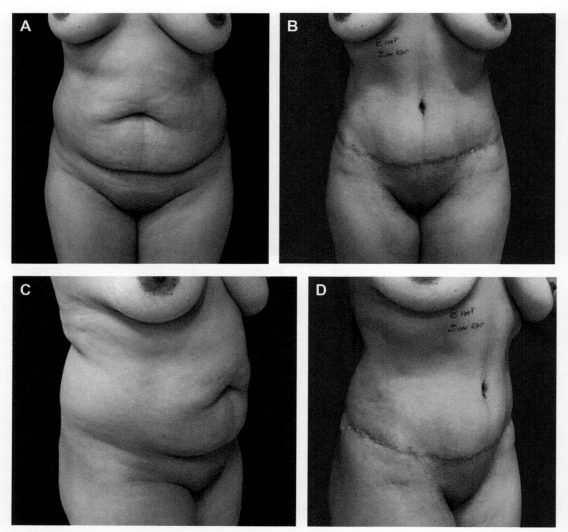

Fig. 18. Clinical case. A 38-year-old patient, BMI of 27, good skin quality, and moderate muscular development. (*A*) Frontal view, preoperative. (*B*) At 18 months postoperative. (*C*) Oblique view, preoperative. (*D*) At 18 months postoperative.

and colleagues[28] 42%, Floros and Davis[29] 34.6%, Van Uchelen and colleagues[30] 29.4%, Neamen and Hansen[31] 37.4%, Stewart and colleagues[32] 18% of early complications) and transverse modified abdominoplasty or abdominoplasty with V-pattern of dissection (Chaouat and colleagues[33] 32%, Hensel and colleagues[34] 32%, Heller and colleagues[28] 17%, Kryger and colleagues[35] 11.1%) with LAP (Heller and colleagues[28] 9%, Samra and colleagues[39] 4.3%, Saldanha and colleagues[5] 0.3%) and have shown the lesser percentage of complications with these techniques. Local complications of traditional abdominoplasty include skin necrosis (1.5%–6.7%), seroma (5%–17.6%), cellulitis (2%–9.2%), dehiscence (7.2%–

10.7%), hematoma (5.4%–5.8%), and revision rate (24.8%–46%).[19–28] This is compared with LAP, where skin necrosis had 0% to 0.9%, seroma had 0.1% to 2%, cellulitis from 0.1% to 2.4%, dehiscence had 0.8% to 2.6%, hematoma had 0.8% to 5.8%, and revision rate had 5% to 10.7%.[28–44] A systemic review published by Xia and colleagues[40] proves the safety of LAP compared with traditional abdominoplasty, involving 14,061 patients with statistically fewer complications in the LAP group (relative risk, 0.85; 95% confidence interval, 0.74–0.97; $P = .017$).

It is clear that, when more perforator vessels are kept on the abdominal flap, the vasculature is more robust and the combination with liposuction does not diminish patient safety.

LAP with anatomic definition means a more aggressive and intense liposuction to achieve a desired result on abdominal contour, which may diminish the lateral vascular contributions to central and distal abdominal flap, which is why preservation of the central perforators of the rectus abdominis muscle can guarantee excellent perfusion and prevent complications.

Liposuction has had an important evolution.[45–53] All the techniques have become more superficial and more artistic, achieving better definition of the abdominal curvatures and musculature sometimes at impressing detailing level. Among all studies, the work of Hoyos and colleagues[6–8] published as "dynamic definition" and "high definition" were the most inspiring and changed our perception about these techniques. One of the first authors that published about abdominal definition with traditional liposuction was Mentz and coworkers[54] in 1993, with a publication that named "abdominal etching" technique, which has evolved to the use of power-assisted liposuction but without ultrasound-assisted liposuction and independent from abdominoplasty because of the risk of combining the two procedures according to the authors.[54–56]

The definition of the abdominal area creates a better result, but when increased risk of flap suffering or high rate of secondary procedures exists,[8] it is our preference to maintain a selective, less aggressive liposuction without compromising the anatomic safety of the landmarks mentioned. It is our belief that caution needs to be taken in some areas of the abdomen to guarantee safety to these procedures that are increasing in popularity, but that must be carefully planned in combination with LAP.

Every patient is different, and they should be anatomically marked to obtain an individualized definition. This concept has changed the classical safety areas of liposuction, leaving the superior and central area of the flap (between the rectus muscles and over point A of the markings, see **Fig. 3**B) as a safe liposuction area and leaving just as a risky area the more distal and central area of the flap, under the new position of the umbilical pedicle (yellow area of the marking, **Figs. 3**B and **4**A). That is why the different areas of liposuction should be used, to diminish trauma in all of the abdominal flap, mainly in the rectal muscle "red" area and the distal "yellow" area of the flap; by doing that, we have maintained the same low rates of complications. These markings were obtained from the work of Hoyos and coworkers[8] and modified to bring safety when performed with LAP.

When anatomic definition is done, it is important to understand that not every patient achieves high definition; in fact, most obtain moderate or even low definition, which depends on BMI, skin quality, and the musculature.

When the musculature is not developed and the patient with appropriate BMI wants to be defined the rectus abdominus fat transfer LAP is an interesting idea that could be used in selected cases.[57]

SUMMARY

The LAP technique is known worldwide, it is safe and reproducible, has low complication rates, and effectively enhances body contour. The new concept of LAP with anatomic definition has shown benefits and improvements on aesthetics results without compromising the safety of traditional LAP. The more natural results of anatomic abdominal definition is a next step in abdominal contour refinement.

DISCLOSURE

All authors have nothing to disclose. No funding was received for this article.

REFERENCES

1. Callia VEE. Dermolipectomia abdominal. São Paulo (MA): Carlo Erb; 1963.
2. Carreirão S, Correa WE, Dias LC, et al. Treatment of abdominal wall eventrations associated with abdominoplasty techniques. Aesthet Plast Surg 1984;8(3):173–9.
3. Saldanha OR, Pinto EB, Matos WN Jr, et al. Lipoabdominoplasty without undermining. Aesthet Surg J 2001;21(6):518–26.
4. Saldanha OR, Federico R, Daher PF, et al. Lipoabdominoplasty. Plast Reconstr Surg 2009;124:934–42.
5. Saldanha OR, Azevedo SF, Delboni PS, et al. Lipoabdominoplasty: the Saldanha technique. Clin Plast Surg 2010;37(3):469–81.
6. Hoyos AE, Perez ME, Castillo L. Dynamic definition mini-lipoabdominoplasty combining multilayer liposculpture, fat grafting, and muscular plication. Aesthet Surg J 2013;33(4):545–60.
7. Hoyos AE, Millard JA. VASER-assisted high-definition liposculpture. Aesthet Surg J 2007;27(6):594–604.
8. Hoyos A, Perez ME, Guarin DE, et al. A report of 736 high definition lipoabdominoplasties performed in conjunction with circumferential Vaser liposuction. Plast Reconstr Surg 2018;142(3):662–75.
9. Tourani SS, Taylor GI, Ashtom MD. Scarpa fascia preservation in abdominoplasty: does it preserve

the lymphatics ? Plast Reconstr Surg 2015;136(2): 258.

10. Friedman T, Coon D, Kanbour-shakir A, et al. Defining de lymphatic system of the anterior abdominal wall: an anatomical study. Plast Reconstr Surg 2015;135(4):1027–32.

11. Har-Shai L, Hayun Y, Barel E, et al. Scarpa fascia and abdominal wall deep adipose compartment preservation in abdominoplasty: current clinical and anatomical review. Harefuah 2018;157(2):87–90.

12. Costa-Ferreira A, Marco R, Vásconez L, et al. Abdominoplasty with Scarpa fascia preservation. Ann Plast Surg 2016;76(Suppl 4):S264–74.

13. Costa-Ferreira A, Rebelo M, Silva A, et al. Scarpa fascia preservation during abdominoplasty: randomized clinical study of efficacy and safety. Plast Reconstr Surg 2013;131(3):644–51.

14. Costa-Ferreira A, Rebelo M, Vásconez LO, et al. Scarpa fascia preservation during abdominoplasty: a prospective study. Plast Reconstr Surg 2010; 125(4):1232–9.

15. Ardehali B, Fiorentino F. A meta-analysis of the effects of abdominoplasty modifications on the incidence of postoperative seroma. Aesthet Surg J 2017;37(10):1136–43.

16. Seretis K, Goulis D, Demiri EC, et al. Prevention of seroma formation following abdominoplasty: a systematic review and meta-analysis. Aesthet Surg J 2017;37(3):316–23.

17. Correia-Gonçalves I, Valença-Filipe R, Carvalho J, et al. Abdominoplasty with Scarpa fascia preservation: comparative study in a bariatric population. Surg Obes Relat Dis 2017;13(3):423–8.

18. Xiao X, Ye L. Efficacy and safety of Scarpa fascia preservation during abdominoplasty: a systematic review and meta-analysis. Aesthet Plast Surg 2017; 41(3):585–90.

19. Nahai F, Brown RG, Vasconez LO. Blood supply to the abdominal wall as related to planning abdominal incisions. Am Surg 1976;42(9):691–5.

20. Huger WE Jr. The anatomic rationale for abdominal lipectomy. Am Surg 1979;45(9):612–7.

21. Boyd JB, Taylor GI, Corlett R. The vascular territories of the superior epigastric and the deep inferior epigastric systems. Plast Reconstr Surg 1984;73:1.

22. Taylor GI, Palmer JH. The vascular territories (angiosomes) of the body: experimental study and clinical applications. Br J Plast Surg 1987;40:113.

23. Taylor GI, Watterson PA, Zelt RG. The vascular anatomy of the anterior abdominal wall: the basis for flap design. Perspect Plast Surg 1991;5:1.

24. El-Mrakby HH, Milner RH. The vascular anatomy of the lower anterior abdominal wall: a microdissection study on the deep inferior epigastric vessels and the perforators branches. Plast Reconstr Surg 2002; 10915:39–47.

25. Rozen WM, Ashton MW, Le Roux CM, et al. The perforator angiosome: a new concept in the design of deep inferior epigastric artery perforator flaps for breast reconstruction. Microsurgery 2010;30:1.

26. Matarasso A, Matarasso DM, Matarasso EJ. Abdominoplasty: classic principles and technique. Clin Plast Surg 2014;41(4):655–72.

27. Smith LF, Smith LF Jr. Safely combining abdominoplasty with aggressive abdominal liposuction based on perforator vessels: technique and review of 300 consecutive cases. Plast Reconstr Surg 2015; 35(5):1357–66.

28. Heller JB, Teng E, Knoll BI, et al. Outcome analysis of combined lipoabdominoplasty versus conventional abdominoplasty. Plast Reconstr Surg 2008; 121:1821–5.

29. Floros C, Davis PK. Complications and long-term results following abdominoplasty: a retrospective study. Br J Plast Surg 1991;44:190.

30. Van Uchelen JH, Werker PMN, Kon M. Complications of abdominoplasty in 86 patients. Plast Reconstr Surg 2001;107:1869.

31. Neamen KC, Hansen JE. Analysis of complications from abdominoplasty: a review of 206 cases at a university hospital. Ann Plast Surg 2007;58(3):292–8.

32. Stewart KJ, Stewart DA, Coghlan B, et al. Complications of 278 consecutive abdominoplasties. J Plast Reconstr Aesthet Surg 2006;59(11):1152–5.

33. Chaouat M, Levan P, Lalanne B, et al. Abdominal dermolipectomies: early postoperative complications and long-term unfavorable results. Plast Reconstr Surg 2000;106:1614.

34. Hensel JM, Lehman JA Jr, Tantri MP, et al. An outcome analysis and satisfaction survey of 199 consecutive abdominoplasties. Ann Plast Surg 2001;46:357.

35. Kryger ZB, Fine NA, Mustoe TA. The outcome of abdominoplasty performed under conscious sedation: six-year experience in 153 consecutive cases. Plast Reconstr Surg 2004;113(6):1807e17.

36. Friedman T, O'Brien Coon D, Michaels V, et al. Fleur-de-lis abdominoplasty: a safe alternative to traditional abdominoplasty for the massive weight loss patient. Plast Reconstr Surg 2010;125:1525–35.

37. Coon D, Gusenoff JA, Kannan N, et al. Body mass and surgical complications in the postbariatric reconstructive patient: analysis of 511 cases. Ann Surg 2009;249:397–401.

38. Levesque AY, Daniels MA, Polynice A. Outpatient lipoabdominoplasty: review of the literature and practical considerations for safe practice. Aesthet Surg J 2013;33(7):1021–9.

39. Samra S, Sawh-Martinez R, Barry O, et al. Complication rates of lipoabdominoplasty versus traditional abdominoplasty in high-risk patients. Plast Reconstr Surg 2010;125(2):683–90.

40. Xia Y, Zhao J, Cao DS. Safety of lipoabdominoplasty versus abdominoplasty: a systematic review and meta-analysis. Aesthet Plast Surg 2018. https://doi.org/10.1007/s00266-018-1270-3.

41. Lázaro CC, Victor LB. Full abdominoplasty with circumferential lipoplasty. Aesthet Surg J 2007; 27(5):493–500.

42. Cárdenas-Camarena L. Aesthetic surgery of the thoracoabdominal area combining abdominoplasty and circumferential lipoplasty: 7 years' experience. Plast Reconstr Surg 2005;116(3):881–90 [discussion: 891–2].

43. Matarasso A. Liposuction as an adjunct to a full abdominoplasty revisited. Plast Reconstr Surg 2000; 106(5):1197–202 [discussion: 1203–5].

44. De Souza Pinto EB, Indaburo PE, Da Costa Muniz A, et al. Superficial liposuction: body contouring. Clin Plast Surg 1996;23(4):529–48.

45. Fodor PB, Cimino WW, Watson JP, et al. Suction assisted lipoplasty: physics, optimization, and clinical verification. Aesthet Surg J 2005;25:234–46.

46. Gasparotti M. Superficial liposuction for flaccid skin patients. Ann Int Symp Recent Adv Plast Surg 1990; 90:441.

47. Gasparotti M. Superficial liposuction: a new application of the technique for aged and flaccid skin. Aesthet Plast Surg 1992;16:141–53.

48. Gasperoni C. MALL liposuction: the natural evolution of subdermal superficial liposuction. Aesthet Plast Surg 1994;18:253–7.

49. Gasperoni C. Rationale of subdermal superficial liposuction related to the anatomy of subcutaneous fat and the superficial fascial system. Aesthet Plast Surg 1995;19:13–20.

50. Wall SH Jr, Lee MR. Separation, aspiration, and fat equalization: SAFE liposuction concepts for comprehensive body contouring. Plast Reconstr Surg 2016; 138(6):1192–201.

51. Jewell ML, Fodor PB, de Souza Pinto EB, et al. Clinical application of VASER-assisted lipoplasty: a pilot clinical study. Aesthet Surg J 2002;22:131–46.

52. Rohrich RJ, Beran SJ, Di Spaltro F, et al. Extending the role of liposuction in body contouring with ultrasound-assisted liposuction. Plast Reconstr Surg 1998;101:1090–102.

53. Gutowski KA. Evidence-based medicine: abdominoplasty. Plast Reconstr Surg 2018;141(2):286e–99e.

54. Mentz HA 3rd, Gilliland MD, Patronella CK. Abdominal etching: differential liposuction to detail abdominal musculature. Aesthet Plast Surg 1993;17: 287–90.

55. Agochukwu-Nwubah N, Mentz HA. Abdominal etching: past and present. Aesthet Surg J 2019. https://doi.org/10.1093/asj/sjz153.

56. Husain TM, Salgado CJ, Mundra LS, et al. Abdominal etching: surgical technique and outcomes. Plast Reconstr Surg 2019;143(4):1051–60.

57. Danilla S. Rectus abdominis fat transfer (RAFT) in lipoabdominoplasty: a new technique to achieve fitness body contour in patients that require tummy tuck. Aesthet Plast Surg 2017;41(6):1389–99.

Drainless Abdominoplasty Using Progressive Tension Sutures

Todd A. Pollock, MD*, Harlan Pollock, MD

KEYWORDS

• Abdominoplasty • Tummy tuck • Drain-free abdominoplasty • Quilting sutures

KEY POINTS

- The goal of this chapter is to give clear and in-depth detail to allow a surgeon to incorporate Progressive Tension Sutures (PTS) into their practice.
- Specifically, a detailed technical description of PTS placement is included with helpful tips to decrease time, dimpling and frustration for those new to the technique.
- Complete details of the authors drain-free abdominoplasty technique using progressive tension sutures including post-operative care, pain management, compression and early activities for improved the patient's experience.
- Details of an in-continuity umbilical inset for a natural appearing neo-umbilicus.
- Criticisms of PTS such as dimpling and increased operative time are addressed with clear suggestions on eliminating these as barriers to using this technique.

DRAINLESS ABDOMINOPLASTY USING PROGRESSIVE TENSION SUTURES

Demand for abdominoplasty continues to grow as bariatric surgery becomes more common, adding to those seeking body contouring for medical weight loss and post-partum abdominal changes. Because of this increase, many changes have been seen in abdominoplasty, improving safety and aesthetics. As a group, surgeons tend to be relatively conservative and slow to change surgical techniques that they either learned in training or have used successfully over many years in practice. This is especially true when that change is something that previously has been considered essential to the operation. And so it is with the use of drains in abdominoplasty. To many plastic surgeons the suggestion of eliminating drains in abdominoplasty is nothing short of sacrilege. From a patient's perspective dread drains preoperatively, find them uncomfortable and burdensome postop, and remember them as the worst part of the abdominoplasty experience. Additionally the use of drains still result in a significantly high rate of seromas adding to office time and expense as well as patient inconvenience and negative experiences.

Today there are several abdominoplasty techniques that promote eliminating drains while decreasing or maintaining seroma rates relative to traditional methods.[1–5] It seems, however, that seroma prevention should start with an understanding of the cause of seroma in abdominoplasty. Although still debated, common theories include excessive dead space, interruption of lymphatic function, and flap motion leading to repeated interference in the healing process. The authors believe that it is this latter theory of motion that contributes most to seroma formation in abdominoplasty, as the strong and multidirectional movement of the abdomen repeatedly disrupts nascent healing. This repeated disruption

Private Practice, 8305 Walnut Hill Lane Suite #210, Dallas, TX 75231, USA
* Corresponding author.
E-mail address: tap@drpollock.com

Clin Plastic Surg 47 (2020) 351–363
https://doi.org/10.1016/j.cps.2020.03.007
0094-1298/20/© 2020 Elsevier Inc. All rights reserved.

leads to increased inflammation and generation of the inflammatory exudate found in abdominoplasty seromas.[6] Secure fixation of the 2 wound surfaces provided by progressive tension sutures allows for uninterrupted healing, which minimizes inflammation and fluid production.

Progressive tension sutures (PTS) are sutures that securely affix a flap in its advanced position over multiple points to the underlying tissue. In abdominoplasty, the sutures are placed from the superficial fascia of the flap to the muscle fascia (**Fig. 1**). These sutures act not only to secure the flap to the underlying tissue to prevent disruption with abdominal motion but also close dead space (**Fig. 2**) and broadly distribute tension over the entire flap.

The authors' experience in using this method preceede the original paper by decades with documentation found in operative notes dating back to 1980. The technique has evolved significantly over time in order to make it more consistent and reproducible. The authors first published the concept of PTS and its use in abdominoplasty to reduce the rate of seromas while eliminating drains in 2000.[3] Since publication of that small consecutive series, the authors updated technical modifications and reviewed their experience in 597 consecutive patients.[5] They also published papers using PTS in facelift, browlift, and latissimus dorsi donor site. But few good ideas develop in isolation, and others have described similar techniques with comparable results.[7,8]

The goal of this article is to describe the technical details of placement of PTS in the context of the authors' abdominoplasty procedure in adequate detail to allow a surgeon to incorporate the use of PTS into their practice.

In addition, they review common barriers surgeons have noted in adding PTS to abdominoplasty and provide ways to avoid these problems. They also review evidence of the effectiveness of PTS in abdominoplasty and support the elimination of suction drains while decreasing the rate of seroma formation.

SURGICAL TECHNIQUE

The primary focus of this article is to provide the surgeon with the technical detail that will allow them to begin to use the progressive tension suturing technique in their abdominoplasties successfully and with as little frustration as the learning

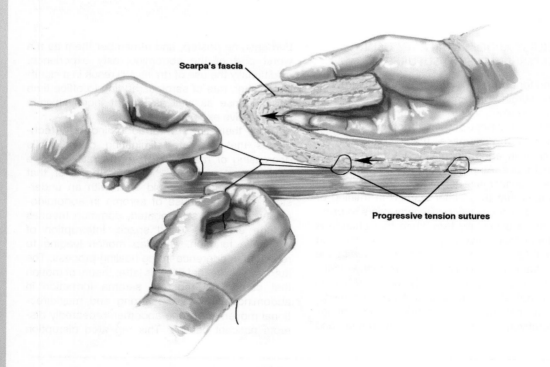

Scarpa's fascia

Progressive tension sutures

Fig. 1. Illustration of PTS placement. Note the suture in the flap must include Scarpa's fascia and muscle fascia for secure fixation. (*From* Pollock TA, Pollock H. Progressive Tension Sutures in Abdominoplasty: A Review of 597 Consecutive Cases. Aesthet Surg J. 2012;36(6):729-742; with permission.)

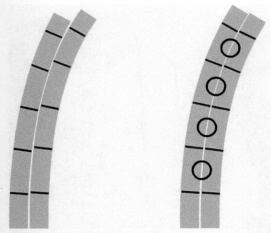

Fig. 2. Graphic diagram illustrates the relationship of the abdominal wall and the abdominal flap with motion. The circles represent progressive tension sutures. Left: there is no fixation and the 2 surfaces shift relative to each other. Right: compared with where the 2 surfaces are fixed and the surfaces move together as a unit.

curve will allow. The authors also detail their general approach to abdominoplasty to share with the reader what they have found to be successful. But, by no means is this protocol meant to be a recipe that requires exact duplication for success. It is very important to understand that PTS is a technical adjunct that can be applied to most abdominoplasty techniques as well as other procedures that involve an advancement flap.

Patient Selection

All patients are assessed for their overall health, surgical risk, and specific indications for body contouring. Patients older than 50 years or with significant health issues are referred to their primary care physician or an appropriate specialist for preoperative clearance and any specific perioperative recommendations for that patients' individual medical condition.

Body mass index (BMI) is considered in assessing a patient's appropriateness for abdominoplasty, and the association of higher BMIs with the increase in complications is respected. But a specific BMI is not considered an absolute contraindication. Patients are evaluated on an individual basis, as well-developed musculature and large bone structure affect BMI negatively without the associated surgical risks seen in obesity. In individuals deemed too great a surgical risk, care is taken to explain their unacceptably risk and a referral to a weight loss specialist is made.

Body contouring procedures on patients who have had a bariatric procedure and lost a significant amount of weight are delayed until weight has been stable for at least 6 months. Patients who have lost weight through diet and exercise over a slower period may be operated on after only 3 months of stable weights if their diet is not one of high caloric restrictions. A nutritional assessment is done in all weight loss patients.

Venous thromboembolic (VTE) risk is assessed using Caprini's identified risk factors and prophylaxed based on these risk factors.[9] All patients have sequential compression devices placed before induction and are ambulated early postoperatively. Chemoprophylaxis is reserved for patients considered high VTE risk and in those who show poor postoperative advancement in ambulation. Subcutaneous enoxaparin is started approximately 8 hours postop for a 7-day course. The patients are ambulated early postop in an upright position. The goal is to ambulate the patient in an upright posture 4 hours following surgery completion. Although considered a VTE risk, compressive garments are used in most cases. More details will be addressed in the section discussing postoperative care. As a final word on this topic, it seems clear that the science of VTE prevention is incomplete and surgeons must rely on their best judgment based on the knowledge available.

Patients who smoke are encouraged to stop but are not strictly required to do so in most instances. The patient is engaged in a candid discussion about smoking's effects on wound healing, VTE, and pulmonary risks and the conversation is documented. A patient's unwillingness to cease smoking is factored into their overall risks, and a determination is made on that patient's acceptability as a surgical candidate. In the authors' series, 13.7% of patients admitted to smoking and those patients had no greater incidence of complications.[5]

Preop Prep and Markings

Patients are marked in an upright position denoting anatomic landmarks, areas of adiposity, and any special considerations such as a lap band port, scars, contour irregularities, or other characteristics of relevance. Areas of adiposity are marked topographically. The incision is marked on the table, as it has been noted that when marked standing it can be displaced superiorly when the patient is placed supine on the table.

The one exception is patients who are having an extended or circumferential procedure in which some excision must be done in a prone position and later joined with the anterior excision. In this case, the anterior- and posterior-lateral excision is planned and marked with the patient standing. The patient is then placed supine and a mark is made at the farthest posterior point along the incision that can be easily worked on from a supine position. This is typically around the midaxillary line or a little posterior. An ellipse is then designed with the posterior excision that ends near that point marked. This marks what will be excised while the patient is in a prone position. Cross-hatching is helpful in aligning the wound edges after excision, and these can be marked at this point or on the table.

Approximately three-quarters of the patients are operated under general anesthesia. The patients are warmed preoperatively in the holding area, and sequential compression devices are applied and begun immediately on entering the operating room. If a concomitant breast procedure is planned, the breasts are not included in the abdominal prep to allow for forced air warming of the upper body while the abdomen is addressed. If available, a bed-warmer is useful in maintaining patient's temperature.

The patient is initially placed prone on the operating table if posterior liposuction or excision is indicated. In most patients some posterior liposuction is used to achieve a good flank contour and rounding of the superior buttocks. The areas to be suctioned (and excised) are infiltrated with wetting solution containing epinephrine only (Lactated Ringers 1 L, 1:1000 epinephrine 1 mL). Local anesthetic adds nothing to the patient under general anesthesia, and it is feared that when liposomal bupivacaine is used, the pooled lidocaine may have a detrimental effect of premature freeing the bupivacaine from the liposomes even after the recommended wait of 20 minutes. The authors infiltrate at approximately a 1:1 ratio with what is anticipated to be removed or as a superwet infiltration. In most cases, the authors choose to infiltrate by hand for more even distribution and for better control of the volume.

When the patient is turned to a supine position the abdomen is marked. Markings are made denoting the incision, approximate area to be excised, costal margin, iliac crest, and approximate lateral rectus (**Fig. 3**). This helps direct liposuction and areas to avoid over defatting based on their postoperative position on the flap. The incision is designed in a gentle curvilinear shape. The central incision over the mons pubis is relatively flat and placed 6 to 7 cm above the vulvar commissure. This measurement and marking need to be done with the mons elevated to the desired postoperative position. The incision is extended at a superiorly directed angle to just

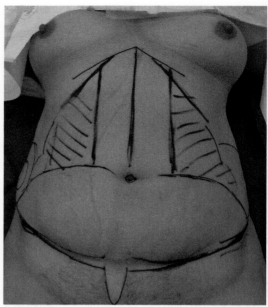

Fig. 3. On the table markings augment the preoperative marking and map out the specific operative plan. First the incision is marked about 7 cm above the vulvar commissure and extended laterally in a curvilinear shape to 1 to 2 cm below the iliac crest. Marking is done with upward tension elevating this tissue to the postoperative level desired. An ellipse is formed with the planned incision marking the anticipated tissue to be excised. A line is marked on either side of midline at the approximate lateral rectus margin. The costal margin and line denoting the angle of the iliac crest are marked creating a triangle with the lateral edge of the rectus. This is the area (cross-hatched) where aggressive liposuction is performed. A circle is sometimes marked (not shown here) just above the umbilicus to represent the tissue that will end up with flap advancement in the lower abdomen. Liposuction is done judiciously here, as it is typically an area of convexity in the attractive female abdomen. If further fat removal is needed after the flap is advanced, it can be done at that time.

below the anterior superior iliac spine. Again, this should be marked while elevating the lower inguinal tissues to their desired postoperative height. The planned incisions are infiltrated with 0.25% Bupivicaine with epinephrine and the areas of liposuction as well as dissection are infiltrated with the same epinephrine-only wetting solution previously described for vasoconstriction and hydrodissection.

In most patients, the greatest amount of liposuction is done in the lateral abdomen and anterior flanks. Liposuction is used as needed under the abdominal flap and in adjacent areas to achieve the desired aesthetic appearance based on individual patient assessment. The authors use liposuction in most of the patients. Their published series documented 67% of patients[5] having suction in the flank and abdomen. Suctioning done under the abdominal flap is limited to the subscarpal plane. The authors use their variation of SAFE liposuction technique[10] with the power-assisted liposuction device in all cases. A 5.0-mm basket cannula is used without suction followed by suctioning with a 5.0-mm double Mercedes cannula. The "equalization"

portion of the SAFE liposuction technique is often omitted.

The authors elevate the abdominal flap with the electrocautery on a cut/coagulation blend and attempt to stay a few millimeters above the muscle fascia leaving a small amount of areolar tissue. Elevation is at that level over the entire abdomen without attempt to preserve Scarpa's fascia. The exception is at the level of the incision, between the lateral Mons and the iliac crest where a cuff of superficial fascia is developed to suture later

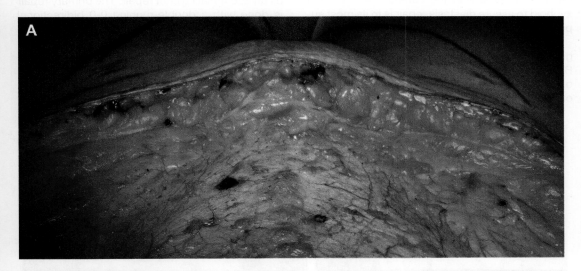

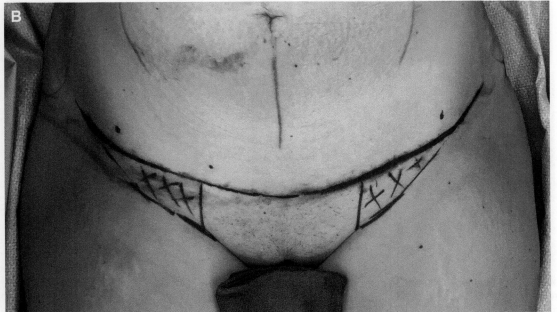

Fig. 4. (*A*) Well-developed edge of Scarpa's fascia. (*B*) Area marked with an X between lateral mons and iliac crest indicates area at risks lateral femoral nerve entrapment. Leaving a well-developed edge of fascia ensures adequate inclusion of fascia while minimizing risk.

in order to assure inclusion of fascia in closure while avoiding a deeper suture bite in this area. This minimizes risk of lateral femoral cutaneous nerve entrapment or irritation (**Fig. 4**). Although electrocautery dissection has been implicated in seroma formation and preservation of Scarpa's fascia has been touted as a means to decrease seroma risk, the authors have had no problems maintaining a very low seroma rate with this technique. The degree of dissection is individualized but wide dissection to the costal margin is most common. Dissection above the costal margin is rarely used except in the central area over the xyphoid to assure diastasis repair is to its most superior extent.

Once dissection is completed to the desired degree, the diastasis recti are marked for repair. Before this repair the fascia is infiltrated generously with 0.25% Bupivacaine with epinephrine or liposomal Bupivacaine 20 cc (266 mg) mixed with 80 cc of 0.25% Bupivacaine with epinephrine as a rectus sheath block and an abdominal wall block or an open TAPS block[11] (**Fig. 5**). Infiltration of this vasoconstrictive solution along the planned rectus repair decreases bleeding of the rectus sheath vessels during the repair.

Interrupted 2-0 PDS sutures are placed at around 3 cm intervals in order to align the rectus repair and take tension off of the running primary closure. In patients with a particularly wide diastasis or poorer fascial quality, these sutures are placed at closer intervals and more completely as an additional layer of repair. The primary repair is done with a double-running 0-0 bidirectional barbed polydioxanone suture. One double strand is started just at the xyphoid and run to the superior aspect of the umbilicus. A second double strand is started just below the umbilicus and run to the pubis. Typically, the goal of the diastasis repair is to simply bring the edges of the rectus

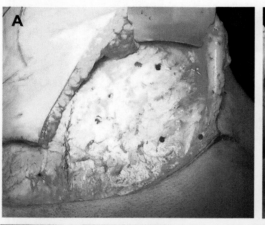
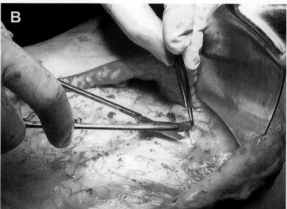
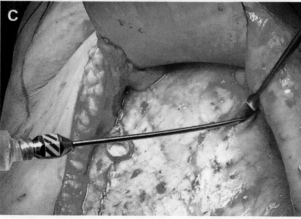

Fig. 5. Open TAPS block. (*A*) Location block is placed 3 cm medial to the anterior superior iliac spine and 9 cm superior. (*B*) The external and internal oblique muscles are split, and the areolar transverses abdominis plane is bluntly dissected. The dissection can be done from the costal margin to the iliac crest. (*C*) A blunt infiltration cannula is used to infuse 10 cc of 0.25% bupivacaine into the space. The muscle split is closed with a single figure of 8 sutures to keep the local anesthetic in the space (not pictured).

muscles together. However, sutures are placed about 1 cm lateral to the muscle edge to account for elasticity of the fascia. Individual cases of secondary repair, extremely wide diastasis, or poor fascial quality may require a greater degree of tightening or the addition of mesh. That discussion is beyond the scope of this article.

Supraumbilical Progressive Tension Suture Placement

The patient is placed in a moderate hip flexed position by putting the head of the bed up to the level that passively advances the abdominal flap to the desired degree, typically about 30 to 45°. The bed is then placed in Trendelenburg until the torso is parallel to the floor. The legs are lowered about 10°. With the use of PTS, less hip flexion is needed, as the sutures powerfully advance the flap on their own. The less hip flexion needed makes PTS placement much easier.

Supraumbilical PTS are only placed in the midline. The authors use 0-0 Vicryl in most patients but 2-0 is adequate in thinner abdominal flaps. Placement of PTS in the supraumbilical abdomen is most efficiently achieved with coordination between the surgeon and the assistant described here for the right-handed surgeon. The surgeon standing on the right side of the table places their left hand behind the highest point of dissection and with their dominant hand places a suture into the flap at that point. The fingers of the nondominant hand can feel as the suture is placed, which helps to assess the depth of placement. It is imperative that the suture includes a good bite of the superficial fascia but not the dermis. The strength of the bite is evaluated by placing tension on the suture. The surgeon's nondominant hand then advances the flap to the desired point on the muscle fascia and the suture is placed in the fascia about 2 cm beyond this point to account for the fascial elasticity. Now the surgical assistant replaces the surgeon's nondominant hand behind the flap and maintains the flap advancement as the surgeon ties the suture (**Fig. 6**). This is repeated about every 2 to 3 cm until the umbilicus is reached, which is around 3 sutures in most cases.

In-continuity Umbilical Inset

Rather than waiting until the abdomen is closed, the umbilicus is inset as the flap is advanced.

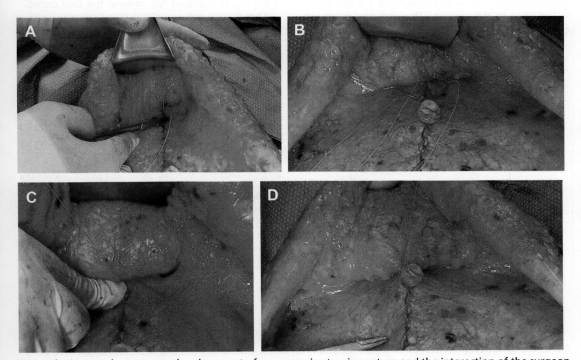

Fig. 6. The images demonstrate the placement of a progressive tension suture and the interaction of the surgeon and the assistant. (*A*) Initially, the surgeon's left (nondominant) hand is behind the flap as the suture is placed, which helps assess depth of placement. (*B*) The flap is advanced to the desired position by the surgeon's left hand, and the suture is placed in the muscle fascia about 2 cm beyond that point. (*C*) The flap is now maintained in the advanced position by the assistant, whereas the surgeon ties the knot. (*D*) Supraumbilical advancement continues until the flap has been advanced to the umbilicus.

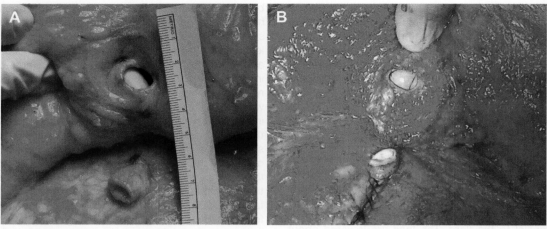

Fig. 7. (*A*) If one examines the abdominal flap in the area of the umbilicus after dissecting the umbilicus free, one will note that there is at least a centimeter rim where there is no fat and just dermis. (*B*) At the site of the umbilical inset, the flap is defatted similarly, which allows the edges of the neoumbilicus to gently curve down in a more natural fashion and brings the suture line into the umbilicus where it is less visible.

This assures that the umbilicus is placed precisely in its native position and allows for a more natural appearance. The umbilical stalk is prepared by trimming it down to a 1 cm circle. On the flap directly above the umbilical stalk, a 2.5 cm circle is defatted to the dermis. The defatted segment of the abdominal flap, which emulates the natural umbilicus (**Fig. 7**), allows the skin to fold downward, creating a natural-looking umbilical shape. A finger is placed in the defatted area and a mark is made on the overlying skin of the flap. A 1 cm circle is marked in the center of the defatted area and excised. The flap is inverted, and additional defatting is done to create an approximately 1 cm rim of defatted flap around the skin defect.

Three-point sutures of 3-0 Vicryl are placed from the deep fascia to the dermal edge of the umbilicus and then to the dermal edge of the abdominal flap and tied down (**Fig. 8**). This is done starting at the 12 O'clock position. The sutures at the 3 and 9

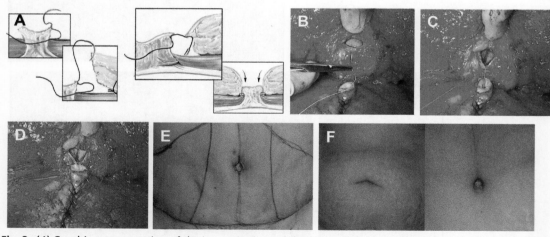

Fig. 8. (*A*) Graphic representation of the in-continuity umbilical inset technique where 3-point sutures are placed between the dermis of the abdominal flap, the dermis of the umbilical stalk, and the muscle fascia to create a more natural-looking umbilicus. (*B, C*) Intraoperative photos of the 12 O'clock suture placement, (*D*) the 3 and 9 O'clock placement, and (*E*) an on-the-table result. Note the gentle curve into the umbilicus with the suture line at the base rather than on the abdominal skin. (*F*) Result preop and year postop. ([*A*] *From* Pollock TA, Pollock H. Progressive Tension Sutures in Abdominoplasty: A Review of 597 Consecutive Cases. Aesthet Surg J. 2012;36(6):729-742; with permission.)

O'clock positions are both placed before tying them down and finally a suture is placed at 6 O'clock position. The effect is to pull the incision (and ultimately the scar) into the depth of the neo-umbilicus. After the abdomen is closed, a few interrupted skin sutures are placed to approximate the skin edges.

Infraumbilical Progressive Tension Suture Placement

Once the umbilicus has been inset, a progressive tension suture is placed just below and then on either side of the umbilicus. From there the central flap is advanced followed by sutures alternating side-to-side to ultimately create a triangular pattern of PTS until the flap is advanced to the distal wound edge (**Fig. 9**). Care is taken to place the sutures symmetrically and with similar tension for even advancement. 0-0 vicryl sutures are placed in the midline, and 2-0 vicryl sutures are used laterally. Typically, about 12 to 15 PTS are placed in total. Minimal assistance is needed on placement of these infraumbilical sutures.

Before the flap is trimmed and inset the mons is first assessed to determine if it needs defatting or superior advancement. Defatting can be done using liposuction or in an open fashion. Defatting in this area should be done conservatively, as over-thinning is undesirable. The Mons should be elevated and secured in an attractive and youthful position. Sutures are placed from the superficial fascia of the Mons to the deep fascia centrally and 3 cm on either side to elevate and secure it at the desired position. Additional sutures may be placed lateral to these if elevation of this area is desired.

The authors cut and inset the flap in the central abdomen just above the Mons first. This central portion of the anterior abdomen is the most visible to the patient and it is the most critical for vascularity. If the umbilical rent cannot be removed, it is converted to a vertical incision. This must be closed in multiple layers including approximation of deep fascia and subcutaneous fat along with the dermis and skin to avoid a visible depression, which may not be noted on the table but appears once the swelling has resolved.

When the flap is trimmed centrally, the dermis is observed for capillary bleeding as a reassuring sign of good vascularity. As the mons area may be thicker than the abdominal flap, care is taken to keep as much fat as is needed on the flap in this area. As the lateral positions of the flap are cut, attention is paid to the thickness of the distal wound edge. The flap is thinned to match the height of where it will be inset with the thinnest areas in the iliac fossa and iliac crest. Scarpa's fascia is often removed for a few centimeters in these thin areas. Three-point sutures of 2-0 vicryl are used between the superficial fascia of the abdominal flap and muscle fascia. Once this is done over the entire incision, the skin edges should gap about 1 cm. The dermis is closed with interrupted 4-0 PTS or vicryl, and the skin is closed with 3-0 polydioxanone bidirectional barbed suture.

Steri-strips are applied to the transverse incision, and antibiotic ointment is applied to the umbilical incision. A lite sterile dressing and a compressive garment are applied. The surgeon will check the binder placement and tightness in the recovery room. Patients are admitted overnight based on the surgeons judgment but in general, if the patient had multiple procedures resulting in a lengthy surgery, if there are significant preexisting medical conditions requiring monitoring, if there was an excessively large amount of tissue resection or liposuction aspirate or electively based on the patient's wishes.

Pain control is based on the concept of multimodal analgesia where several interventions are used to address pain at various points along the pain pathway to minimize or eliminate the use of narcotics. This has been found to be very successful in minimizing narcotic use and improving the patients' experience. Understanding the concept and various protocols of multimodal analgesia or enhanced recovery after surgery[12,13] are beyond the scope of this article but are well worth the readers' time if they are unfamiliar.

The authors' protocol is to use intraoperative bupivacaine or liposomal bupivacaine and a field

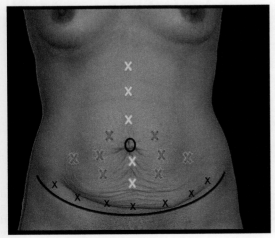

Fig. 9. Typical location and suture type of where progressive tension sutures are placed. This changes with patient size and amount of dissection.

block with or without a TAPS block. They also give intravenous acetaminophen toward the beginning of the procedure and Ketorolac at the end.[14] If the patient stays overnight these drugs are given every 8 hours alternating every 4 hours. This provides excellent pain control with very little need for rescue narcotics. As an outpatient the authors use celecoxib 200 mg every 12 hours. Some recommend starting this the night before surgery, but it has not been found to be necessary. This is taken for the first 2 weeks after surgery. Muscle relaxants are given to patients with wide diastasis repair. Patients are given a small number of a narcotic for breakthrough pain.

Patients are ambulated early and in an upright posture, as the authors are very confident in the secure fixation the PTS provide. The authors' goal is to have the patients ambulate within 4 hours after surgery. They ask the patients to stand as erect as they are comfortable and the majority (more than 60% in an informal patient survey) walks completely upright in the first 24 hours following surgery. They are encouraged to ambulate regularly and with increased frequency as they progress. They are asked to wear the binder or compressive garment as much as possible in the first 2 weeks primarily for comfort but also for edema control. The authors encourage good pulmonary toilet through incentive spirometry and coughing to clear secretions and provide instructions to avoid constipation.

Discussion

Sir Almroth Wright observed that "Every novel idea or new invention must, before it wins general acceptance, pass through three stages. It is, to begin with, repudiated as absurd. After that, is allowed to be reasonable. And, finally, it is belittled as obvious." This is the course the authors have observed in the concept of PTS and their use in drain-free abdominoplasty taking. Having recently noted mention of PTS in abdominoplasty review articles,[15–17] questions on the board recertification review material and the test itself, and the spreading of use into reconstructive literature, the concept seems to be well into the general acceptance stage and on the cusp being considered obvious as a tool to prevent seromas. Yet, there still seems to be some barriers that prevent some surgeons from adopting PTS.

The 2 most common reasons surgeons will attribute for not using PTS in abdominoplasty are concern for permanent dimpling and increased surgical time. A third reason some surgeons suggest as the basis for not using PTS is that they believe they simply do not work.

In regard to dimpling, if PTS are properly placed from the superficial fascia to the muscle fascia it is nearly impossible to get a permanent dimple. One can demonstrate this by placing a suture in the superficial fascia of the abdominal flap and apply tension to that suture while placing the distal flap under tension in an inferiorly directed tension. No matter how hard one pulls on the suture in fascia,

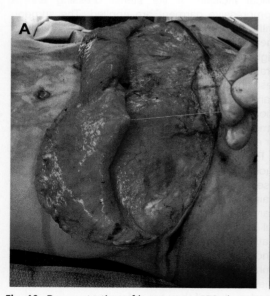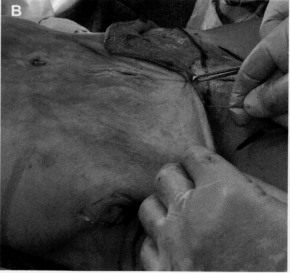

Fig. 10. Demonstration of how proper PTS placement in scarpa's fascia cannot produce a dimple in the skin. (*A*) Suture is placed in Scarpa's fascia, and firm tension is applied. (*B*) Flap is gently advanced inferiorly, and no dimple is seen no matter how hard one pulls on the suture.

no dimple will appear (**Fig. 10**). However, a suture placed too close to or into the dermis will leave a dimple.

There are 2 situations where a temporary dimple or irregularity can appear that may unnecessarily concern a surgeon new to PTS. The first is when a progressive tension suture is properly placed, and the flap is secured in its advanced position. A dimple will form at the spot where the suture is placed defining the transition point of the advance tissue to the lax tissue of the elevated flap. This we have termed the *advancement dimple*. On placement of the next PTS and further advancement of the flap, the previous dimple disappears and a new one is formed at the new transition point between advanced and lax tissue. Discussions with many surgeons initially trying the technique have described repeatedly placing and cutting the PTS on seeing this advancement dimple, fearing that the dimple is permanent. This unnecessary suture replacement adds to the operative time and frustrates the surgeon, often leading them to abandon the technique. The understanding of the concept of the temporary advancement dimple is imperative to avoid these problems.

It may be desirable to advance the abdominal flap in a direction not directly inferior. For example, some may desire to direct the infraumbilical flap from lateral to medial in order to avoid a dog-ear or shorten the incision. Irregularity may also be seen due to lines of tension created in the skin if the vector of pull is not in line with the previous PTS. These lines of tension are temporary and most commonly disappear in 24 hours or less as the skin relaxes. Analogously, plastic surgeons can relate seeing lines of tension following a flap closure of a defect only to find they are gone when the patient returns to the office.

Concern for increased operating time is another common barrier. In the authors' experience, placement of PTS over the entire flap including the inset of the umbilicus typically adds around 20 minutes once the surgeon has gained some experience. This decrease is primarily gained in coordination between the surgeon and the surgical assistant as described earlier in the techniques section. Although the authors have timed their PTS placement for videos and commentaries, no formal studies have been done. It should also be noted that when they began using PTS their goal was to close dead space and they used 30 to 40 sutures.[3] Over time, they have come to realize that secure fixation of the 2 surfaces is the most important and that closure of dead space need not be as complete. Today the authors place 12 to 15 sutures and this alone decreases time.

Other studies have looked at surgical time comparing abdominoplasty with and without PTS, and their results were similar to the authors's experience. Three studies specifically evaluate the difference in operative time of abdominoplasty with and without the use of PTS.[18–20] There was a wide variation in placement times between these studies ranging from 1 to 54 minutes, with the average time being 23 minutes. Rosen[21] and Gutowski[22] have modified the technique to make PTS placement faster by using a running barbed suture in place of the interrupted PTS technique and shown comparable effectiveness in seroma prevention. Unfortunately, neither has formally studied time or time savings. Although the authors' experience and the available studies that have evaluated placement times indicate that the additional time for placement is not excessive, more studies are needed.

A third reason surgeons may choose to not use PTS is that they do not believe that they actually work. A healthy degree of skepticism is reasonable when considering a substantive change to what has been considered in the past a fundamental part of a procedure. However, today the supportive evidence abounds. Numerous papers regarding the PTS in abdominoplasty have been published in multiple forms.

To start, there are several large series (level 4 evidence) that demonstrate significant reduction in seroma when PTS were added to their abdominoplasty. Antonetti[23] reviewed a single surgeon's abdominoplasty experience of 517 patients over a 30-year period. They divided the patients into 5 groups based on significant changes in technique over the years. Their rate of seromas requiring aspiration dropped from 24% in outpatient abdominoplasty with drains to 1.7% with the addition of PTS without drains. Macias and colleagues[24] reviewed their experience of 451 abdominoplasties over a 7-year period performed by multiple surgeons. Their seroma rate showed a statistically significant drop from 9% with drains to 2% when PTS were added. Overall complication rates were similar, and there was no difference when liposuction was added. Sforza and colleagues[25] reviewed 414 abdominoplasties dividing them into 3 groups (D = 100, PTS + D = 226, PTS = 88). They had 12% seromas with drains alone and no seromas in the 314 patients in whom PTS were placed. The presence of drains made no difference.

Randomized controlled studies (level 2 evidence) are limited in aesthetic surgery, and this is true for studies on PTS as well. Jabbour[26] did a systematic literature review looking for randomized controlled trials (RCT) that compared PTS with and without the use of drains and those comparing PTS with or without drains to drains only. They found 3 RCT that met this criterion. Three studies[18,20,27] evaluated PTS (+/− drains) to drains alone and the meta-analysis (which also included some retrospective studies) showed the PTS group to have a significantly lower seroma rate. Comparisons between PTS + drains and PTS alone showed no statistical difference and thus no benefit to adding drains when PTS are used.

In the RCT study by Andrades and colleagues,[18] they showed an equal seroma rate between PTS and drains and their seroma rate in both groups was very high (D = 33%, PTS = 33%, PTS + D = 27% by clinical evaluation). However, their seroma volumes on the first aspiration were low in all groups (D = 45 cc, PTS = 64 cc, PTS/D = 45 cc), and second aspiration volumes were nominal with around 20 cc in each group. Not unexpectedly, ultrasound evaluation showed higher fluid volumes. It also showed compartmentalization of the fluid in the PTS groups, which the authors would suggest make it less clinically obvious and more readily absorbed without need for puncture in the clinical setting.

A meta-analysis done by Ardehali and Fiorentino[28] looked at various abdominoplasty modifications believed to reduce seroma, which included PTS, preservation of Scarpa's fascia, and fibrin glue, whereas the analysis showed statistically significant seroma reduction in both the Scarpa's preservation and PTS groups and not in the fibrin glue group. Risk of bias was considered high due to the high number of retrospective trials.

PTS have been used in several reconstructive procedures, with traditionally high seroma rates adding to the supportive evidence of their effectiveness in preventing seromas. Arguably, no procedure has a higher seroma rate than the latissimus donor site. Rios and colleagues[29] demonstrated the reduction of seroma in the latissimus dorsi donor site from 30% with drains to 0% with PTS and drains in a small retrospective series. Other more recent randomized controlled studies of latissimus donor site confirm significant reduction of seromas, earlier drain removal, and hospital stay.[30,31] Other studies have demonstrated similar advantages in DIEP flap breast reconstruction[32] and abdominal wall reconstruction.[33]

SUMMARY

The abdominoplasty technique described will hopefully serve as a guide for surgeons to incorporate PTS into their practice with as little challenge as possible. It should also serve to eliminate the common fears of dimpling through proper suture placement and reduce time for PTS placement through a practiced coordination between surgeon and assistant. Based on the bulk of the currently available evidence, PTS are an effective means in decreasing seroma in abdominoplasty. Certainly, more high-powered, RCTs are needed to be definitive. These studies also support the concept that the addition of drains in abdominoplasty where PTS are used do not seem to add any benefit and can be safely omitted. Eliminating drains, which are universally disliked by patients, along with early, upright ambulation and multimodal analgesia, improves the patient experience and speed recovery.

DISCLOSURE

The authors have nothing to disclose.

REFERENCES

1. Rodby KA, Stepniak J, Eisenhut N, et al. Abdominoplasty with suction undermining and plication of the superficial fascia without drains: a report of 113 consecutive patients. PlastReconstr Surg 2011; 128:973–81.
2. Epstein S, Epstein M, Gutowsk K. Lipoabdominoplastywithout drains or progressive tension sutures: an analysis of 100 consecutive patients. AesthetSurg J 2015;354:434–40.
3. Pollock H, Pollock T. Progressive tension sutures: a technique to reduce local complications in abdominoplasty. PlastReconstr Surg 2000;105(7):2583–6.
4. Quaba A, Conlin S, Quaba O. The no-drain, no-quilt abdominoplasty: a single-surgeon series of 271 patients. PlastReconstrSurg 2015;135:751–60.
5. Pollock H, Pollock TA. Progressive tension sutures in abdominoplasty: a review of 597 consecutive cases. AesthetSurg J 2012;32:726–44.
6. Andrades P, Prado A. Composition of post-abdominoplastyseromas. AesthetPlast Surg 2007;31(5): 515–8.
7. Mladick R. Progressive tension sutures to reduce complications in abdominoplasty. PlastReconstr Surg 2001;107:619.
8. Baroudi R, Ferreira C. Seroma; how to avoid it and how to treat it. AesthetSurg J 1998;18(6):439–41.
9. Pannucci CJ, MacDonald JK, Ariyan S, et al. Benefits and risks of prophylaxis for deep venous thrombosis and pulmonary embolus in plastic surgery: a systematic review and meta-analysis of controlled trials and consensus conference. PlastReconstr Surg 2016;137:709–30.
10. Wall S, Lee M. Separation, aspiration, and fat equalization: SAFE liposuction concepts for comprehensive body contouring. PlastReconstr Surg 2016; 138(6):1192–201.

11. Fiala T. Tranversusabdominis plane block during abdominoplasty to improve postoperative patient comfort. AesthetSurg J 2015;35(1):72–80.

12. Elias KM. Understanding enhanced recovery after surgery guidelines: an introductory approach. J LaparoendoscAdvSurg TechA 2017;10:1089.

13. Pedziwah M, Kisalewski M, Wierdak M. Early implementation of Enhanced Recovery after Surgery (ERAS) – protocol compliance improves outcomes: a prospective cohort study. Int J Surg 2015; 3(Suppl):S117.

14. Gobble RM, Hoang HLT, Kachniarz B, et al. Ketorolac does not increase perioperative bleeding: a meta-analysis of randomized controlled trials. PlastReconstrSurg 2014;133(3):741–55.

15. Gutowski K. Evidence-based medicine: abdominoplasty. PlastReconstrSurg 2018;141:286e–99e.

16. Shestak K, Rios L, Pollock T, et al. Evidence-based approach to abdominoplastyupdate. AesthSurg J 2019;39(6):628–42.

17. Rosenfield L, Davis C. Evidence-based abdominoplasty review with body contouring algorithm. AesthetSurg J 2019;39(6):643–61.

18. Andrades P, Prado A, Danilla S, et al. Progressive tension sutures in the prevention of postabdominoplastyseroma: a prospective, randomized, double-blind clinical trial. PlastReconstr Surg 2007;120(4):935–46.

19. Khan S, Teotia SS, Mullis W, et al. Do progressive tension sutures really decrease complications in abdominoplasty? Ann Plast Surg 2006;56(1):14–21.

20. Margara A, Boriani F, Granchi D, et al. Is the high superior tension technique an equivalent substitute for progressive tension sutures in post-bariatric abdominoplasty? A comparison prospective study. PlastReconstr Surg 2014;133(3):544–9.

21. Rosen AD. Use of absorbable running barbed sutures and progressive tension technique in abdominoplasty: a novel approach. PlastReconstr Surg 2010;125(3):1024–7.

22. Gutowski KA, Warner JP. Incorporating barbed sutures in abdominoplasty. AesthetSurg J 2013;33(3 Suppl):76S–81S.

23. Antonetti JW, Antonetti AR. Reducing seroma in outpatient abdominoplasty: analysis of 516 consecutive cases. AesthetSurg J 2010;30(3):418–25.

24. Macias LH, Kwon E, Gould DJ, et al. Decrease in seroma rate after adopting progressive tension sutures without drains: a single surgery center experience of 451 abdomniplasties over 7 years. AesthetSurg J 2016;36:1028–35.

25. Sforza M, Husein R, Andjelkov K, et al. Use of quilting sutures during abdominoplasty to prevent seroma formation: are they really effective? AesthetSurg J 2015;35(5):574–80.

26. Jabbour S, Awaida C, Mhawej R, et al. Does the addition of progressive tension sutures to drains reduce seroma incidence after abdominoplasty? A systematic review and meta-analysis. AesthetSurg J 2017;37(4):440–7.

27. Di Martino M, Nahas FX, Barbosa MVJ, et al. Seroma in lipoabdominoplasty and abdominoplasty: a comparative study using ultrasound. PlastReconstr Surg 2010;126(5):1742–51.

28. Ardehali B, Fiorentino F. A meta-analysis of the effects of abdominoplasty modifications of seroma prevention. AsthetSurg J 2017;37(10):1136–43.

29. Rios J, Pollock T, William A. Progressive tension sutures to prevent seroma formation after latissimusdorsi harvest. PlastReconstr Surg 2003;112:1779–83.

30. Hart A, Duggal C, Ximena P, et al. A prospective randomize trial of the efficiency of fibrin glue, triamcinolone acetonide, and quilting sutures in seroma prevention after latissimusdorsi breast reconstruction. PlastReconstr Surg 2017;139(4):854e–63e.

31. Dancey AL, Ceema M, Thomas S. A prospective randomized trial of the efficacy of marginal quilting sutures and fibrin sealant in reducing the incidence of seroma in the extended latissimusdorsi donor site. PlastReconst Surg 2010;125:1309–17.

32. Nagarkar P, Lakhiani C, Cheng A, et al. No-drain DIEPflap donor-site closure using barbed progressive tension sutures. PlastReconstrSurg Glob Open 2016;4:e672.

33. Janis J. Use of progressive tension sutures in component separation: merging cosmetic techniques with reconstructive surgery outcomes. PlastReconstr Surg 2012;130:851–5.

Abdominoplasty with Combined Surgery

Michele A. Shermak, MD

KEYWORDS

- Abdominoplasty • Hernia repair • Lipoabdominoplasty • Lower body lift • Mommy makeover
- VTE prophylaxis • Surgical safety

KEY POINTS

- Abdominal contouring surgery as a combination procedure is common, and driven by deformities resulting from issues that systemically impact individuals, including aging, weight loss, and pregnancy.
- Breast surgery is often performed at the time of abdominoplasty; combining breast surgery and abdominal surgery must take opposing forces of lift into consideration.
- Body lifts including lower back lift and thigh lift are often performed in conjunction with abdominoplasty as a lower body lift for individuals with aged, lax tissues or for individuals who have sustained massive weight loss.
- Combination procedures may be safely performed, with a focus on efficiency in the operating room, limiting blood loss and hypothermia, and attending to potential need for venous thromboembolism prophylaxis.

INTRODUCTION

Abdominoplasty is one of the top 5 cosmetic plastic surgery procedures performed in the United States.[1] Many individuals consult with a plastic surgeon for abdominal contouring needs related to lax, redundant skin, stretch marks, abdominal muscle laxity, umbilical deformities, and unsightly scars. Pregnancies, abdominal surgeries, aging, and significant weight loss are causes for presentation and result in more global contour issues extending beyond the abdomen alone.

Abdominoplasty is therefore often requested and performed in combination with surgery on other body regions. The abdomen serves as a central focal area, stimulating interest in addressing adjacent areas for more global improvement. In our published series of patients undergoing body contouring for weight loss, abdominal improvement was the most prevalent reason for presentation, with 92% of patients in our series undergoing abdominal surgery, often in addition to other procedures.[2] Abdominoplasty may be combined with breast surgery, particularly for women who are post partum, for men with gynecomastia, or for men and women who have sustained massive weight loss through diet or bariatric surgery. Abdominoplasty is also often combined with surgery on the lower back and/or thigh regions, defined as belt lipectomy and lower body lift, for individuals who have lost significant weight or have lax tissues related to aging and sun exposure. Abdominoplasty is most commonly performed with liposuction, including contouring of the back, waist, and upper and lower extremities. Fat transfer to the buttocks and breast has gained increasing popularity in combination with liposuction and abdominoplasty. Abdominoplasty also may be combined with intra-abdominal procedures such as hernia repair and gynecologic procedures.

Liposuction is the procedure most commonly performed in conjunction with abdominoplasty. Lipoabdominoplasty has become increasingly mainstream, with increasingly greater volumes of lipoaspirate proven to be safe.[3] Matarasso[4]

Johns Hopkins Department of Plastic Surgery, Private Practice, 1304 Bellona Avenue, Lutherville, MD 21093, USA
E-mail address: shermakmd@gmail.com

Clin Plastic Surg 47 (2020) 365–377
https://doi.org/10.1016/j.cps.2020.02.001
0094-1298/20/© 2020 Elsevier Inc. All rights reserved.

published the circulation zones of the abdominal skin when liposuction was becoming a more popular adjunct to abdominoplasty in 1995, and this article still serves as a guide to safe liposuction performance in conjunction with abdominoplasty. In more contemporary literature, Saldanha and associates[5] advocate for a more aggressive approach, performing liposuction of the abdominal skin, tolerated by limiting undermining of the skin between the xiphoid notch and umbilicus and with preservation of Scarpa's fascia on the abdominal wall.

Combining cosmetic plastic surgery procedures is appealing. If there are multiple body region concerns, combining surgery allows for 1 recovery period and reduced surgical costs. The overall result can also be appreciated with 1 procedure, improving a more encompassing physical landscape, as opposed to addressing 1 area that is adjacent to another region that, left untreated, takes away from the aesthetics of the overall result. The outcome of combined surgery on adjacent areas is often more than just the sum of the parts, because each area may further enhance adjacent areas (**Fig. 1**). There have been no formal studies on quality-of-life impact with abdominoplasty combination procedures, but it only seems logical that the outcome of safely performed combination procedures is greater than the abdomen treated in isolation. The Body Q outcomes tool will certainly aid in performance of such a study.[6]

More extensive cosmetic plastic surgical procedures are not for everyone. Medical and surgical history must be considered. Medical comorbidities such as diabetes, cardiovascular disease, pulmonary disorders, sleep apnea, morbid obesity, and autoimmune conditions present contraindications to more complicated surgical procedures that present greater challenges to optimal recovery. Tobacco use and vaping also forecast significant healing challenges. Rather than perform combination procedures, staging may be offered to patients presenting with red flags to limit exposure to risk of one larger surgical procedure. Further, hospital-based surgery with overnight observation might be considered over ambulatory surgical center.

Overall optimization of safety is critically important. A surgical team including an experienced anesthesia provider, first assistant, and surgical technician to more expertly aid in exposure and closure help to decrease distractions, shorten procedural duration, and lessen the morbidity of a large multistage surgical procedure. Attention to positioning is critically important to avoid complications associated with nerve compression and stretch, as well as pressure issues, vascular

compromise, and vision. Warming the patient with fluids, blankets, and ambient room temperature decreases the risks of anemia, wound healing issues, and infections. Prophylaxis against venous thromboembolism (VTE) is particularly important in the abdominoplasty procedure given the relatively high incidence reported in the recent plastic surgery literature. A modified Caprini scale helps to guide the choice of providing anticoagulation.[7] Work by Pannucci and associates[8] to more precisely determine the effective dosage of anticoagulants is ongoing. As they have described, a strict daily dosage does not necessarily provide effective prophylaxis for every patient.[8]

TECHNIQUES IN COMBINING ABDOMINOPLASTY WITH OTHER PROCEDURES
Abdominoplasty and Hernia Surgery

Most plastic surgeons have trained in general surgery so they understand basic principles in straightforward hernia repair, taking techniques of plication repair of the rectus diastasis 1 step further. It is not recommended for plastic surgeons with little experience in hernia repair to perform such repairs nor is it advocated that the plastic surgeon approach incarcerated and/or complex hernia presentations if not properly schooled in such techniques. Many times hernias such as umbilical hernias and incisional hernias from laparoscopic procedures are incidentally encountered during what is expected to be a routine abdominoplasty. Repairing hernias while they are exposed assists in best care for the patient, preventing incarceration issues or a more difficult dissection in the future.

It is better to treat umbilical hernias at the time of abdominoplasty rather than at a separate setting, because umbilical hernia repair is particularly problematic if performed before abdominoplasty. As a standalone procedure, umbilical hernias are typically approached by detaching the umbilicus from the abdominal wall, repairing the hernia, sometimes with mesh, then reattaching the umbilicus after repair, leading to decreased circulation from the abdominal wall to the umbilicus. This strategy will not present a problem for later miniabdominoplasty lacking a circumumbilical incision; however, when abdominoplasty requires an incision around the umbilicus, comprising the majority of abdominoplasty cases, circulation to the umbilicus will be totally cut off with incisions under and around the umbilicus. Umbilical hernias are therefore best treated at the time of abdominoplasty. When approaching these hernias, the umbilical stalk may be incised at the most prominent

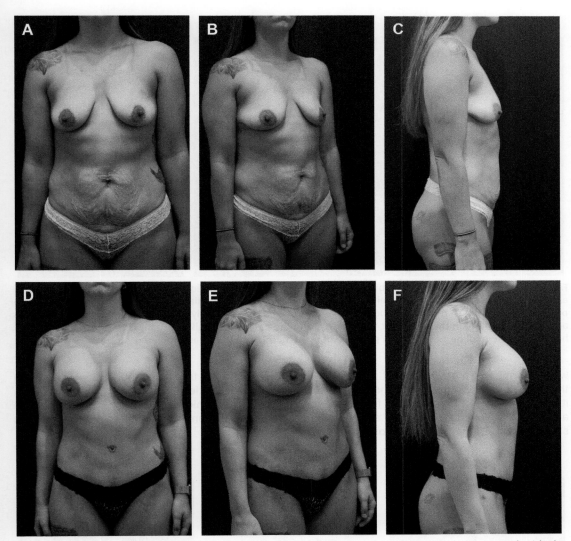

Fig. 1. (*A–C*) Frontal, oblique, and lateral views of a 27-year-old post partum woman who presented with the typical sequelae of pregnancy, including breast deflation and pseudoptosis, and abdominal laxity with stretch marks, lax abdominal muscles, and incongruity at the junction of the pubis and thigh. (*D–F*) Frontal, oblique, and lateral views 8 months after submuscular breast augmentation with silicone gel implants and abdomino-plasty with plication of abdominal muscles and waist liposuction with power-assisted liposuction. Without surgery on her breasts, she would not have had as pleasing a result.

location of the umbilical hernia, allowing entrance into the stalk, reduction of the hernia contents (which is almost always omentum), and closure of the base of the umbilical stalk with permanent suture to block future herniation of the omental fat (**Fig. 2**). The incision on the umbilical stalk is closed and plication of rectus diastasis will then follow.

When encountering incisional and ventral hernias during elevation of the abdominal skin off the abdominal wall, the hernia must be dissected free, with reduction of hernia contents and

approximation of the abdominal wall edges with permanent suture, preferably interrupted figure of 8 sutures to avoid potential unraveling of the hernia repair (**Fig. 3**). In patients with a prior midline incision and underlying ventral hernia, excision of the midline scar and adjacent skin using a fleur-de-lis approach will improve exposure, scar, and contour outcome.

Abdominoplasty and Liposuction

During abdominoplasty, liposuction may be performed on the upper and lower back and lateral

A

B

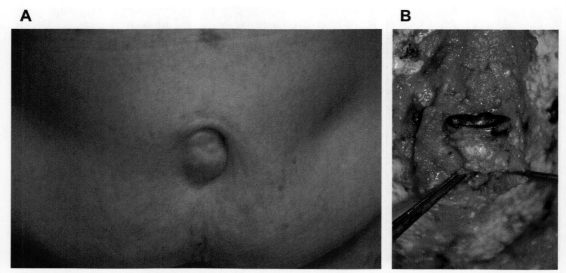

Fig. 2. (*A*) Preoperative photo of umbilicus with a visible hernia. The patient is a candidate for abdominoplasty and her options would have been limited if she underwent umbilical hernia before abdominoplasty. (*B*) Intraoperative photo in which the stalk of the umbilicus was opened longitudinally along the axis of the stalk. With this access, the omentum in the hernia sac was reduced and the base of the stalk internally closed to block recurrent herniation. The midline fascia is then plicated after the hernia is reduced and repaired.

waist to improve circumferential aesthetics of the torso, as long as the patient has good quality skin that would benefit more from deflation and subcutaneous fat reduction, and less from skin removal. Circumferential liposuction takes the result of traditional abdominoplasty to a much higher level, improving and smoothing the waist, flank, and bra line, and creating a sleeker junction with the pubis and upper thigh (**Fig. 4**).

A

B

C

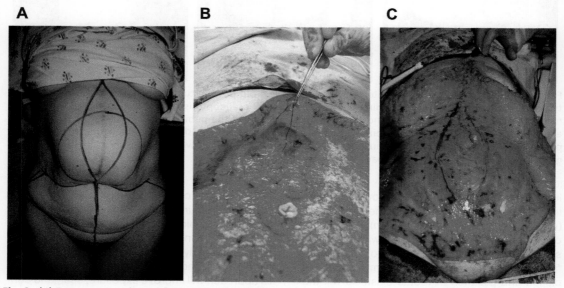

Fig. 3. (*A*) Preoperative photo of a 40-year-old woman who sustained massive weight loss through open gastric bypass surgery. After losing more than 100 lb, she has bulge from ventral hernia and excess abdominal skin. (*B*) After midline elliptical skin excision as marked, the hernia edges are freed, and a loose running Prolene suture from bypass surgery is removed. (*C*) The hernia is primarily fixed, and the rectus abdominal plication will follow in the lower abdomen to adequately reapproximate rectus abdominis muscles from xiphoid to pubis. The skin will be closed as a fleur-de-lis.

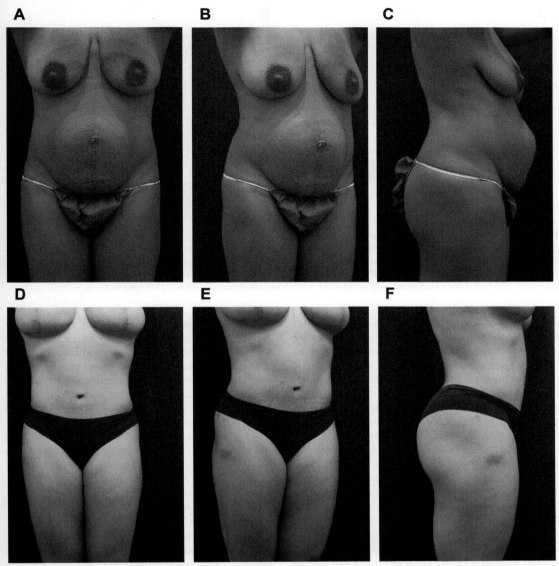

Fig. 4. (*A–C*) Frontal, oblique, and lateral views of a 31-year-old woman who had 4 pregnancies and was left with deflated pseudo ptotic breasts, severe laxity of her abdominal skin and muscles, and loss of shape in her gluteal region. (*D–F*) She is photographed more than a year after her surgery, which included abdominoplasty with muscle repair and mesh reinforcement of her plication, augmentation mastopexy, and liposuction of her back with gluteal fat transfer. This restored her prepregnancy model body.

Intraoperatively, the patient is first positioned prone with careful padding, and positioning of the head and neck and arms so that liposuction may be completed on the back. Careful attention is paid to safe positioning, placing gel rolls under the upper chest/axilla and across the lumbar region. Axillary regions are supported. Arms are positioned perpendicular to the body and at the elbow. Arms and legs are placed on cushioned surfaces. The face should be placed in a prone pillow, avoiding any pressure on the eyes and maintaining the neck in neutral position. Sequential compression devices are in place and active throughout the surgery (**Fig. 5**). Fat grafting to the buttocks might also be performed at that time if indicated.

The patient is then turned supine. Before starting the abdominoplasty, tumescent solution is infused to the waist to allow the hemostatic effect of the solution to work. Abdominoplasty is then

A **B**

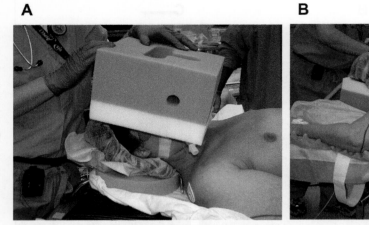

Fig. 5. (*A*) After intubation, the patient has protective eye goggles and prone pillow placed in preparation for prone positioning. (*B*) In the prone position, multiple protective measures have been taken. The neck is in neutral. There are gel rolls, one under the sternum supporting the axillary regions, and the other across the lumbar region. Arms and elbows are positioned at 90° to avoid traction on nerves. The patient is well-padded and warmed. She has a foley catheter and sequential compression devices in place and functioning.

performed, and liposuction of the waist and hip takes place after skin removal and temporary closure of the abdominal wound to allow adequate time for hemostatic effect of the tumescent solution. Augmented liposuction technologies such as power-assisted liposuction or ultrasound-assisted liposuction (vibration amplification of sound energy at resonance) create smoother results than traditional suction-assisted lipectomy.

Although liposuction of adjacent areas improves aesthetic outcome of abdominoplasty, liposuction may also be performed in other areas to improve patient satisfaction. Such areas include the neck, arms, and lower extremities. The surgeon must be mindful about potential blood loss, operating room time, systemic hemodynamic effects associated with greater amounts of liposuction, and protection against VTE. Volume limits are not rigidly set and publications demonstrate safety with greater amounts of lipoaspirate.[3]

Abdominoplasty and Breast Surgery

Patients often desire combining surgery of the abdomen and chest. The breast and abdomen are adjacent and viewed in continuity, so the lack of surgery on one of these areas may detract from the results of surgery on the other area. Individuals most apt to pursue combination abdomen and breast surgery include men with gynecomastia, men with massive weight loss leading to excess skin of the chest with ptotic nipple position, and women who are post partum or who have sustained massive weight loss with deflation and sagging of their breasts. In men with straightforward

gynecomastia requiring liposuction and subareolar gland removal, there is no impact between the chest and abdomen that will impair results at either site. Conversely, when chest skin reduction and management of the breast crease come into play with breast lift, breast reduction, breast augmentation, and gynecomastia procedures in men with significant skin excess from massive weight loss, forces involved in improving the abdomen and chest might work against each other. Vectors of tension required to lift the chest oppose those needed to tighten the abdomen, so these opposing vectors of pull may negatively impact outcome, resulting in poor contours, thickened scars, and/or wound healing problems.

The inframammary fold (IMF) descends with weight loss and with aging. IMF descent is also common with macromastia. In combined abdominal and breast surgical procedures, this author advocates for performing breast surgery first. If abdominoplasty is performed before breast surgery in patients with descent of the IMF, breast aesthetics are more apt to be negatively impacted by abdominoplasty before setting the crease. With suspension of the IMF in breast reduction or lift with either vertical or Wise pattern approaches or in breast augmentation, not only is the breast crease set, but also a secondary reverse abdominoplasty results. This upper abdominal lift actually improves the results of the abdominoplasty, addressing the highest region of the abdomen that might not be adequately addressed from the inferior approach of the standard abdominoplasty (**Fig. 6**).

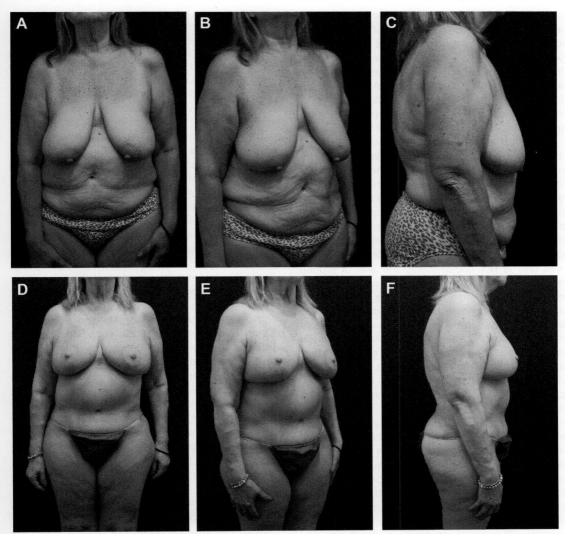

Fig. 6. (*A–C*) Frontal, oblique, and lateral views of a 62-year-old woman who presented with severe ptosis of her breasts with descent of her IMF, as well as significant abdominal muscle and skin laxity. She has significant abdominal deformity with a high umbilicus with skin excess above and below. (*D–F*) Frontal, oblique, and lateral views after breast reduction with inferior pedicle and Wise pattern, with abdominoplasty with muscle plication and waist and back liposuction with power-assisted liposuction. She is photographed 10 months after surgery. Setting her breast fold helps secondarily to elevate the upper abdomen, enhancing the aesthetics of her overall result.

Setting the IMF in breast procedures requires suturing of the deep Scarpa's fascia of the upper abdominal skin flap, or superficial fascial system as described by Lockwood[9], to the breast skin flaps. A 3-way permanent suture further stabilizes the incision placement to the chest wall. With breast augmentation, particularly with larger profile implants, when using an IMF approach fixing the crease by suturing the deep fascia of the lower aspect of the incision to the chest wall with permanent sutures avoids distortion of the crease or bottoming out of the implant when combined with opposing tension associated with the abdominoplasty.

Abdominoplasty and Lower Back Lift

Abdominoplasty and lower back lift comprise the belt lipectomy. This procedure is effective for individuals who have sustained significant weight loss, or for thin, athletic individuals who are body conscious and dissatisfied with lax tissues unresponsive to exercise. Abdominoplasty without addressing the back skin in individuals with significant skin excess and laxity will lack optimal outcome in their body lift procedure, leaving them with excess hip tissue, outer thigh laxity, and buttock ptosis and deflation. A back lift performed in conjunction with abdominoplasty provides more than the sum of its parts, creating global lift and reduction of the lower torso.

Belt lipectomy must be marked with the patient standing. The abdominoplasty marks are connected to the back markings, allowing for lift of lax outer thigh skin, bowing out the markings at the junction area between the back and abdomen laterally at the hip. Conversely, planned skin excision in the midback is minor, because the skin in this location is adherent and typically less redundant. The back midline also does not suffer tension well and is not uncommonly the site of wound healing issues. To minimize risk, a conservative excision is marked in the midline of the back, and the excision may be tailored and increased as a V in the mid upper gluteal cleft once safe tension is determined after excision of the back tissue is completed and the wound is temporarily approximated. Cross-hatch marks are also recommended within back markings to help guide closure and avoid bringing a dogear into the abdomen (**Fig. 7**).

When performing belt lipectomy, a foley catheter is placed to carefully monitor hemodynamics and fluid status. Prone procedure is performed first. Safe prone positioning precautions are followed. A back lift is most safely performed with tailor tacking technique, creating the upper incision and dissecting inferiorly toward the buttock, leaving a layer of lymphovascular fascial tissue over the deep muscular fascia that will later aid in reduction of seromas and edema development. More tissue may be maintained on deep fascia to allow for autoaugmentation of deflated buttocks. In cases of more severe gluteal deflation, flaps based on the superior and inferior gluteal arteries may be designed to augment gluteal fullness. The aesthetics of the back closure are aided by careful tailoring of the midline as a V to guide perception of a more optimal gluteal shape. Drains should be placed to minimize risk of seroma. Tissue glue is placed on the incision closure to seal it and ease dressings.

The patient is then carefully turned supine onto a roller placed on a stretcher and the patient is transferred back to the operating table. Abdominoplasty is then performed with careful tailoring of the lateral junction region between the back and abdomen, completing the belt lipectomy.

Abdominoplasty and Thigh Lift

Abdominoplasty or belt lipectomy optimize the outcome of a thigh lift by providing upward forces of tension that secondarily benefit thigh positioning, particularly in weight loss patients. A thigh lift is performed after the lower back lift because the back lift elevates the buttocks and infragluteal crease directly, and the thighs indirectly, so that markings may need to be adjusted downward for the planned thigh lift. Similarly, abdominoplasty is performed before the anterior thigh lift, because secondary lift of the thigh occurs. A thigh lift may either be performed proximally circumferentially as in the anterior proximal extended thigh lift, or as a vertical extended thigh lift classically performed for massive weight loss patients.[10,11] The anterior proximal extended thigh lift is this author's preferred approach for patients undergoing belt lipectomy because the impact of the thigh lift is compounded by the back lift, and the incisions are well-hidden in bathing suits and underwear. Patients with good skin quality and skin redundancy to the upper half of the thigh have excellent results with lower body lift using the anterior proximal extended thigh lift (**Fig. 8**).

The prone portion of the surgery starts first, with the lower back lift. After the lower back lift is done, infragluteal marking might need to be placed lower for the thigh lift, and the posterior portion of the thigh lift proceeds, removing a hemicrescent of skin at the infragluteal crease, maintaining deep fascia over the hamstring muscles, and fixing the skin up to the ischial periosteum to fix the infragluteal crease.

The patient is then turned supine, completing the abdominoplasty first, followed by completion of the anterior portion of the thigh lift. If a vertical thigh lift is planned, this is done in the anterior position after abdominoplasty is completed.

Abdominoplasty and Gynecologic Procedures

Abdominoplasty performed in conjunction with the gynecologic service requires a collaborative effort in terms of staging, positioning the patient, and determining the best approach for intra-abdominal access for the gynecologist, while also working together to manage a safe postoperative recovery. The patient should be marked by the plastic surgeon preoperatively. Although typically the gynecologist operates first, ideally the plastic surgeon will be present at the beginning of the case to assist the gynecologist in access using incisions planned for the abdominoplasty, possibly creating the incisions to ensure the plan for abdominoplasty is not thwarted by

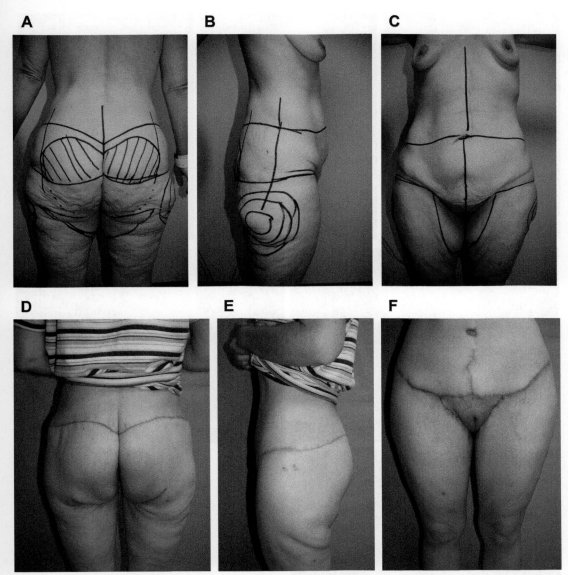

Fig. 7. (*A–C*) Preoperative markings of the back, side, and abdomen of a 40-year-old woman for a circumferential lower body lift. Markings are also present in preparation for autologous gluteal augmentation flaps and anterior proximal extended thigh lift. On the back, hatch marks are created to guide approximation of the closure intraoperatively. Planned skin excision is far less on the midback relative to the outer thigh, as the markings flare from medial to lateral. (*D–F*) Postoperative photos were taken 2 months after surgery. She has global improvement in her torso and thigh regions provided by the circumferential approach.

incision markings disappearing during the gynecologic procedure. Once the gynecologic portion of the procedure is done, the abdomen undergoes a second sterilizing preparation and requires a new table of instruments to combat potential postoperative infection and wound healing problems. The plastic surgeon should be engaged in early postoperative care to optimize healing. Postoperative VTE anticoagulation prophylaxis may need to be introduced with a longer surgery or procedures that increase the VTE risk score. Conversely, anticoagulation may not be advisable from a plastic surgery perspective, but routinely implemented by the gynecologist, so this factor should be discussed with the gynecologist to determine the safest plan to balance minimization of VTE risk with the risk of undesired hematomas.

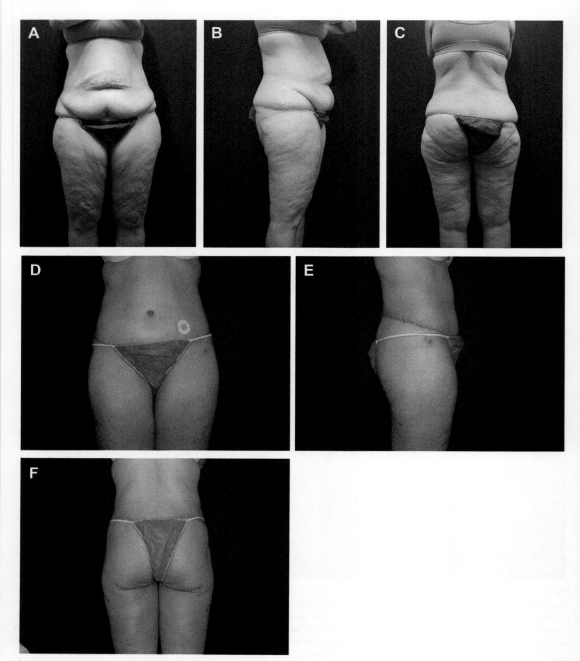

Fig. 8. (*A–C*) This 50-year-old woman presented after massive weight loss from bypass performed through upper transverse abdominal incision. She had lax skin and muscle of her abdomen, thighs, and back, with deflation. (*D–F*) She is photographed 9 months after lower body lift. The belt lipectomy enhances the impact of the hidden incision in the anterior proximal extended thigh lift.

DISCUSSION

Combining plastic surgery of multiple body regions including the abdomen has been a subject of great interest in the literature. Much of the literature has focused on outcomes, with a primary focus on safety and risk of complications, including VTE risk.

Matarasso and Smith[12] shared their experience combining abdominoplasty with cosmetic breast surgery, in addition to performing a review of their own practice and a review of the literature. They found it was more common than not in their practice to combine abdominoplasty with an additional procedure. They did not believe that any specific alterations were necessary in performing abdominoplasty in combination with breast surgery because they believe that the abdomen and breast are 2 distinct regions that do not impact each other. They did not alter their approach to the breast procedure (augmentation, reduction, mastopexy, or augmentation/mastopexy) when combining it with abdominoplasty. They endorse combining breast and abdominal surgery, placing important safety measures into practice.

Chaput and colleagues[13] responded to this paper in a Letter to the Editor, citing their review of the literature of abdominoplasty combined with breast procedures. They found that, of 4 relevant studies, 2 studies determined significantly elevated risk of major complications when combining abdominoplasty and breast surgery, with odds ratios of 5.35 and 14.71. Major complications included death, VTE, cardiac events, flap necrosis, need for transfusion, and infection. Chaput and colleagues disagreed, as this author does, that the abdomen and breasts are distinct body regions that do not impact the other, citing problems with IMF positioning in breasts requiring lowering of the fold, as well as wound healing issues of inverted T incisions owing to tension from the abdominoplasty in combined breast abdominal procedures. One suggestion they posit is to stage the abdomen and breast into 2 separate procedures.

Looking at body lift procedures for weight loss patients, Coon and colleagues[14] found that performing multiple procedures in the same operative setting increases the total number of complications for a given number of trips to the operating room, but the absolute number of complications was no greater than would be expected if all procedures had been performed individually.

Vieira and colleagues[3] studied more than 11,000 patients who underwent abdominoplasty with (n = 9638 [86.1%]) and without (n = 1553 [13.9%]) truncal liposuction within the Tracking Operations and Outcomes for Plastic Surgeons database and actually found a decreased risk of seroma and overall complications (10.5%) when adding liposuction to abdominoplasty procedures when performed by board-certified plastic surgeons. The reduced risk was theorized to be related to careful surgical technique with limited undermining. Furthermore, volumes of lipoaspirate corresponding to 100 mL per unit of body mass index did not confer an increased risk of morbidity in this study. This finding is particularly interesting and informative because states like Florida have mandated

limits to the amount of liposuction performed at the time of abdominoplasty, based on no concrete data.

Pereira and Sterodemus[15] studied their patients undergoing abdominoplasty combined with liposuction of the back and fat transfer to the buttock or thigh. In their database of 64 consecutive patients with over an average follow-up of 3 years, they found a 5% risk of early complications, including infection and hematoma, with a 14% prevalence of late complications, including scarring and contour deformities. Appearance was self-reported to be very good to excellent in 63% of their patients. The authors concluded that there was high patient satisfaction with a single operation combining abdominoplasty with liposuction and gluteal fat grafting.

As reported by Winocour and colleagues,[16] who used the CosmetAssure database to assess outcomes, combining procedures with abdominoplasty increased the risk of complications. The complication risk of abdominoplasty alone was 3.1%, whereas adding procedures increased overall risk: liposuction, 3.8%; breast procedure, 4.3%; liposuction and breast procedure, 4.6%; body contouring procedure, 6.8%; and liposuction and body-contouring procedure, 10.4%. These authors concluded that combined procedures can significantly increase complication rates and should be considered carefully in higher risk patients.

CosmetAssure data are limited in that outcomes are only captured if patients self-report. Saad and colleagues[17] were able to capture data from California Office of Statewide Health Planning and Development Ambulatory Surgery Database and reliably track 477,741 patients from the outpatient setting to the inpatient setting from 2005 to 2010 without relying on self-reported data. Patient medical history, hormone use, previous pregnancy, and hypercoagulable conditions were described as well. The authors found some combinations of elective outpatient procedures conferred an additive, and sometimes more than additive, VTE risk. Although combining 2 procedures did not confer a greater risk of 30-day hospital admission, emergency department visit, or mortality rates, the authors found that VTE risk had a greater than additive 30-day and 1-year risk with concurrent abdominoplasty and liposuction, and a greater than additive 1-year risk with concurrent abdominoplasty and hernia repair.

Hatef and colleagues[18] performed a meta analysis literature review investigating VTE risk with procedures combined with abdominoplasty. Thirty papers qualified to provide data for their analysis, which demonstrated that the highest rates of

VTE followed circumferential abdominoplasty at 3.40% and abdominoplasty combined with an intraabdominal procedure at 2.17%, relative to VTE rates of abdominoplasty alone at 0.35% and abdominoplasty with concomitant plastic surgery at 0.79%.

Iribarren-Moreno and colleagues[19] studied combining abdominoplasty with obstetric procedures. They found that the morbidity of abdominoplasty increases when performed in combination with obstetric procedures. There is a high risk of infections, thrombosis, and skin necrosis, and sometimes fatal VTE. Furthermore, aesthetic outcome is less assured with risk of redundant skin, unsatisfactory scars, abdominal wall defects, poor contour, and unaddressed skin folds when combining abdominoplasty with obstetric procedures. Ali and Essam[20] found that combining abdominoplasty with cesarean section led to higher complication rates and inferior aesthetic results secondary to distorted local anatomy and compromised healing because of contamination. Voss and colleagues[21] demonstrated higher morbidity, longer operative times, and protracted hospital stays when abdominoplasty was combined with common gynecologic operations. In this study, 6.6% of patients undergoing combined procedures had a pulmonary embolism, versus no patients undergoing a single procedure.

The literature is replete with studies looking at large existing datasets of patients undergoing abdominoplasty combined with other procedures. More commonly, these studies are identifying complications with emphasis on VTE outcomes. There are currently no papers in the literature presenting prospective data on patients undergoing these combined procedures. Further, there are no data on aesthetic outcomes or quality-of-life indicators. With a validated instrument available, BodyQ, plastic surgeons are well-positioned to conduct this type of study in the future.

SUMMARY

There is a great societal appeal for abdominal combined surgical procedures. Abdominoplasty is one of the most sought after cosmetic plastic surgery procedures, and consultation for abdominoplasty serves as a gateway to discussing extension of contour outcome and amplification of aesthetic outcome by adding surgery on other body regions. Combination surgery has become the norm and more common that isolated abdominoplasty in many practices, with an appeal that is galvanized by lower costs and one recovery period. Attention to the impact of surgery on body regions adjacent to the abdomen is important, and regional lifts serve to help or hinder outcomes, depending on tension forces that work in concert or opposition. Surgical planning must take patient factors into consideration, particularly those that will challenge healing and recovery. Staging and hospital-based surgery are alternatives that may need to be incorporated into surgical planning. VTE risk and avoidance has become the most studied variable in these combination procedures. VTE is the most common poor outcome and is particularly important because it may be fatal. Strategies have been discussed to minimize this risk as well as others, while also optimizing aesthetic results.

DISCLOSURE

There are no commercial or financial conflicts of interest or any funding sources to report.

REFERENCES

1. Available at: https://www.plasticsurgery.org/documents/News/Statistics/2018/plastic-surgery-statistics-full-report-2018.pdf. Accessed March 17, 2020.
2. Shermak MA, Chang D, Magnuson TH, et al. An outcomes analysis of patients undergoing body contouring surgery after massive weight loss. Plast Reconstr Surg 2006;118(4):1026–31.
3. Vieira BL, Chow I, Sinno S, et al. Is there a limit? A risk assessment model of liposuction and lipoaspirate volume on complications in abdominoplasty. Plast Reconstr Surg 2018;141(4):892–901.
4. Matarasso A. Liposuction as an adjunct to a full abdominoplasty. Plast Reconstr Surg 1995;95(5):829–36.
5. Saldanha OR, Azevedo SF, Delboni PS, et al. Lipoabdominoplasty: the Saldanha technique. Clin Plast Surg 2010;37(3):469–81.
6. Reavey PL, Klassen AF, Cano SJ, et al. Measuring quality of life and patient satisfaction after body contouring: a systematic review of patient-reported outcome measures. Aesthet Surg J 2011;31(7):807–13.
7. Pannucci CJ, Barta RJ, Portschy PR, et al. Assessment of postoperative venous thromboembolism risk in plastic surgery patients using the 2005 and 2010 Caprini Risk score. Plast Reconstr Surg 2012;130(2):343–53.
8. Pannucci CJ, Fleming KI, Bertolaccini C, et al. Double-blind randomized clinical trial to examine the pharmacokinetic and clinical impacts of fixed dose versus weight-based enoxaparin prophylaxis: a methodologic description of the fixed or variable enoxaparin (FIVE) trial. Plast Reconstr Surg Glob Open 2019;7(4):e2185.

9. Lockwood T. Reduction mammaplasty and masto-pexy with superficial fascial system suspension. Plast Reconstr Surg 1999;103(5):1411–20.

10. Shermak MA, Mallalieu J, Chang D. Does thigh-plasty for upper thigh laxity after massive weight loss require a vertical incision? Aesthet Surg J 2009;29(6):513–22.

11. Mathes DW, Kenkel JM. Current concepts in medial thighplasty. Clin Plast Surg 2008;35(1):151–63.

12. Matarasso A, Smith DM. Combined breast surgery and abdominoplasty: strategies for success. Plast Reconstr Surg 2015;135(5):849e–60e.

13. Chaput B, Bertheuil N, Alet JM, et al. Combined ab-dominoplasty and breast surgery versus isolated abdominoplasty: results of a systematic review. Plast Reconstr Surg 2016;137(1):248e–9e.

14. Coon D, Michaels JV, Gusenoff JA, et al. Multiple procedures and staging in the massive weight loss population. Plast Reconstr Surg 2010;125:691–8.

15. Pereira LH, Sterodimas A. Composite body contour-ing. Aesthet Plast Surg 2009;33(4):616–24.

16. Winocour J, Gupta V, Ramirez JR, et al. Abdomino-plasty: risk factors, complication rates, and safety of combined procedures. Plast Reconstr Surg 2015;136(5):597e–606e.

17. Saad AN, Parina R, Chang D, et al. Risk of adverse outcomes when plastic surgery procedures are combined. Plast Reconstr Surg 2014;134(6): 1415–22.

18. Hatef DA, Trussler AP, Kenkel JM. Procedural risk for venous thromboembolism in abdominal contouring surgery: a systematic review of the literature. Plast Reconstr Surg 2010;125(1):352–62.

19. Iribarren-Moreno R, Cuenca-Pardo J, Ramos-Gallardo G. Is plastic surgery combined with obstet-rical procedures safe? Aesthet Plast Surg 2019; 43(5):1396–9.

20. Ali A, Essam A. Abdominoplasty combined with ce-sarean delivery: evaluation of the practice. Aesthet Plast Surg 2011;35:80–8.

21. Voss SC, Sharp HC, Scott JR. Abdominoplasty com-bined with gynecologic surgical procedures. Obstet Gynecol 1986;67:181–5.

Noninvasive Abdominoplasty

Dennis J. Hurwitz, MD*, Lauren Wright, DO

KEYWORDS

- VASER • BodyTite® • Morpheus8® • Radiofrequency micro needling • Liposuction • UAL
- Ultrasonic assisted lipoplasty • Abdominoplasty

KEY POINTS

- New energy-based technologies may supplant invasive surgery for mild to moderate skin laxity.
- New energy based technologies may reduce the extent of surgery and resulting scars.
- Access to effective and safe energy based technologies provides a wide range of options for consumers interested in noninvasive and minimally invasive techniques.
- New energy based technologies can have a reasonable return on investment by increasing referrals for traditional body-contouring procedures.

 Video content accompanies this article at http://www.plasticsurgery.theclinics.com.

INTRODUCTION

For decades in the senior author's practice, the most frequent aesthetic surgery request has been for improvement of abdominal contour. Patient presentations vary from thin with wrinkles to obese with a hanging pannus and oversized girth. Additionally, patients are frequently concerned with oversized flanks and backs, and sagging mons pubises and buttocks. Once surgical options, which involve removal of excess skin and fat, are discussed, patients' responses range from abhorrence to surgery and/or scars to acceptance of whatever incisions it takes to obtain the desired result. Most inquirers for contouring of the torso not only welcome but are intrigued by noninvasive and minimally invasive treatments to supplant or augment anticipated or revision abdominoplasty.

Patients readily grasp that in the process of correcting their abdominal contour deformities, their entire torso can be recontoured. To obtain the optimal result, the authors favor oblique flankplasty and lipoabdominoplasty supplemented with ultrasonic assisted liposuction, radiofrequency skin tightening, and electromagnetic energy muscular enhancement.

Comprehensive contouring of the torso involves up to 8 interactive tools. Complex and lengthy excisions are complimented with preoperative weight reduction and intraoperative energy-based technologies.

1. *Human choriogonadotropin (HCG)/500 calorie a day diet* to reduce high body mass index[1,2]
2. *VASER* ultrasound-assisted lipoplasty to debulk fat, undermine flaps, and harvest adipose tissue[3,4]
3. *BodyTite* bipolar radiofrequency to tighten subcutaneous tissue[5]
4. *Morpheus8* bipolar radiofrequency to tighten and rejuvenate skin[6]
5. *Lower body lift* with abdominoplasty when flank laxity is absent
6. *Oblique flankplasty with lipoabdominoplasty (OFLA)* to narrow a sagging waist, tighten the torso, and lift the buttocks and lateral thighs[7]
7. *J Torsoplasty with breast reshaping* to compliment an OFLA or lower body lift[8]

Hurwitz Center for Plastic Surgery, 3109 Forbes Avenue, #500, Pittsburgh, PA 15213, USA
* Corresponding author.
E-mail address: drhurwitz@hurwitzcenter.com

Clin Plastic Surg 47 (2020) 379–388
https://doi.org/10.1016/j.cps.2020.03.005
0094-1298/20/© 2020 Elsevier Inc. All rights reserved.

8. *EmSculpt* high-frequency electromagnetic energy for muscular development and toning[9]

This article now focuses on noninvasive and minimally invasive energy-based treatments that supplant, minimize, or compliment abdominoplasty. For optimal delivery of patient care and to stay competitive, plastic surgeons should embrace appropriate supportive technologies.

Nonplastic surgeons often working in noncertified clinics and spas are usurping patients through marketing of energy-assisted technologies for improved abdominal contour. Their message is that advanced, expensive technology offers scarless, painless, rapid recovery and a safer alternative to abdominoplasty. Having only 1 or 2 machines, these clinics are tempted to expand their limited therapeutics beyond the appropriate indications. Given their depth of training in traditional body contouring techniques, plastic surgeons are in the best position to provide quality care using these newer technologies. This is clearly in the best interest of our patients. Based on our conscientious effort to sift through competing manufacturers' claims and clinical cases, this article presents the technology we

have chosen and how we apply it into our patients concerned about their torso aesthetics.

EXTERNAL APPLICATION OF ENERGY (SculpSure, TruSculpt)

The most popular noninvasive application of energy is the external freezing of adipose. Aware of the saturation of Coolsculpt machines in the Pittsburgh market, and its occasional side effect of paradoxic adipose hypertophy, we have purchased both the laser (SculpSure) and radiofrequency (TruSculpt) alternatives. Our TruSculpt from Cutera is too new to comment on. However, the Hurwitz Center has about an 80% patient satisfaction in more than 50 patients with using SculpSure. The set of three 20-minute applications of the penetrating CO_2 laser with immediate skin cooling requires mild sedation, while obtaining subtle improvements. We have had no incidences of paradoxic adipose hypertrophy in our small series.

Frustrated body builders have an alternative to enhancing strength and tone to both core and extremity muscles (**Fig. 1**). We are applying EmSculpt to early postoperative abdominoplasty and VASERlipo patients and have seen encouraging

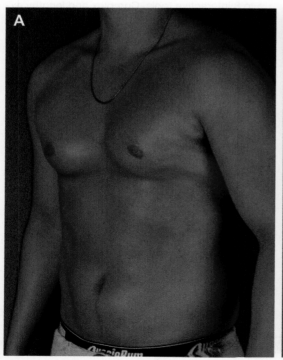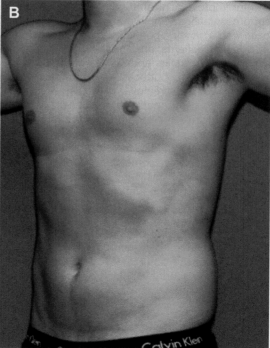

Fig. 1. The effect of EmSculpt on a muscular 27-year-old man. (*A*) Pretreatment left anterior oblique view of the torso. (*B*) Three months after four 40 minute applications of EmSculpt shows mild decrease in subcutaneous adipose and increased muscular definition of the rectus abdominus muscles.

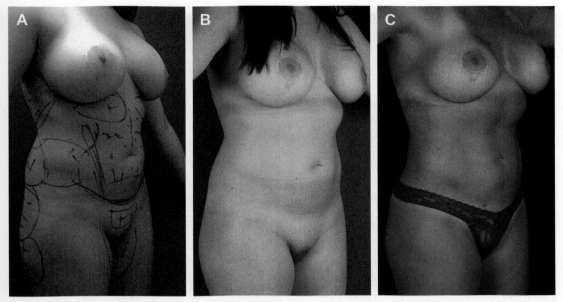

Fig. 2. Combining VASERlipo with BodyTite for a minimally invasive abdominoplasty in a 27-year-old overweight woman, along with VASERlipo of her flanks and saddlebags and lipoaugmentation of her lateral gluteal areas. Three months later, she underwent 4 EmSculpt high-frequency electromagnetic energy treatments. Right Oblique views. (*A*) Presenting condition with preoperative markings for VASERlipo, BodyTite. (*B*). Presenting condition without surgical markings. (*C*) Four months after, she has a smoothly sexy proportional and naturally muscular appearance.

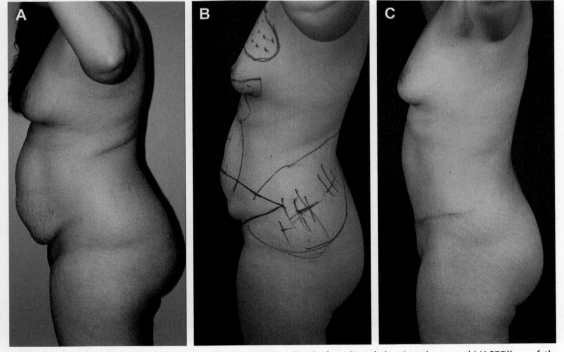

Fig. 3. Reduction of obesity with HCG/500 calorie a day diet before lipoabdominoplasty and VASERlipo of the flanks as seen on left lateral views. (*A*) Presentation of 32-year-old woman with a body mass index of 31 for abdominoplasty and repair of the diastasis recti. (*B*) After a loss of 30 pounds, the patient is marked for lipoabdominoplasty and VASERlipo of the flanks. Notable is the reduction of abdominal protuberance and absence of back rolls. (*C*) Two years after her lipoabdominoplasty, VASERlipo of the flanks and 150 mL lipoaugmentation of the breasts.

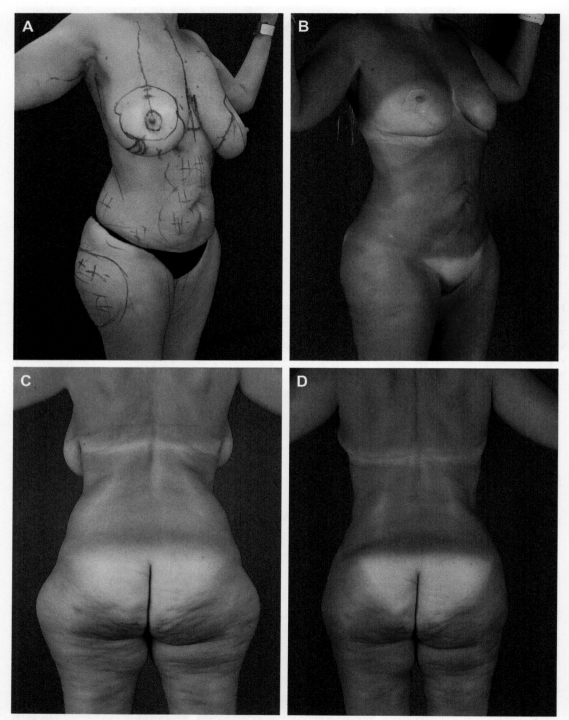

Fig. 4. Combining VASERlipo with BodyTite for a minimally invasive abdominoplasty, and reduction of saddle-bags, medial thighs, and flanks in a 64-year-old woman having a circumvertical, superior pedicle beast reduction. (*A*) Before. (*B*) Six months after (right anterior oblique view). (*C*) Before. (*D*) Six months after (posterior view). Her abdomen, medial thighs, and saddlebags were both bulging with adipose and lax skin; hence the VASERlipo followed by BodyTite, except for the flanks which did not have loose skin. After images show complete resolution of her saddlebags and medial thigh bugles without loose skin. Her generalized wavy loose abdominal skin is being treated with Morpheus8.

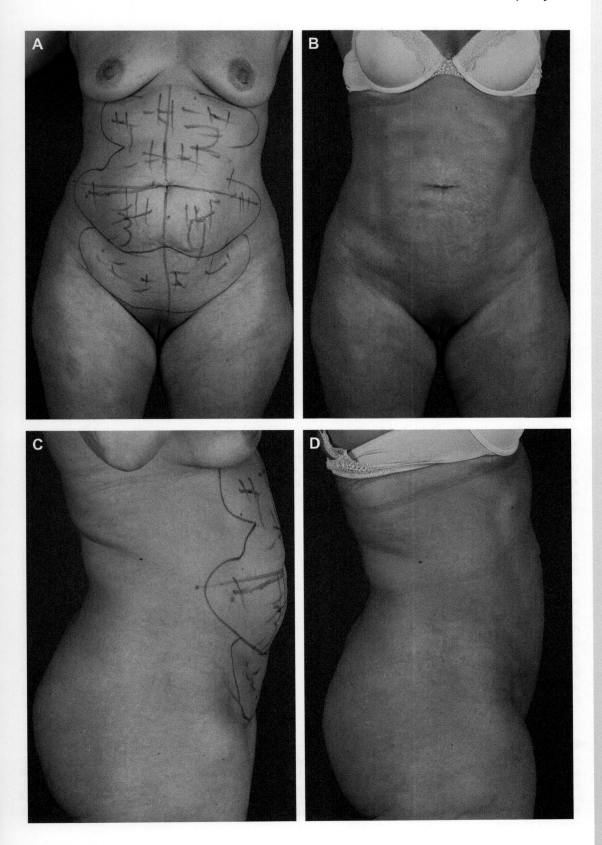

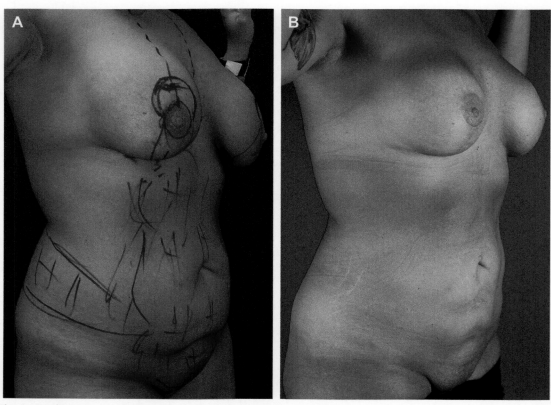

Fig. 6. Combining VASERlipo with BodyTite for a minimally invasive abdominoplasty in a 32-year-old with depression superior to her ptotic mons pubis and VASERlipo of her flanks. The surgeon performed implant exchange and Wise pattern mastopexies, while assistants performed the minimally invasive surgery. (*A*) Before presenting condition with presurgical markings for the mastopexies and VASERlipo and BodyTite of anterior abdominal wall and VASERlipo of her flanks and (*B*) 6 months after right anterior oblique images. She has a "gap" deformity that has annoying adipose-laden skin laxity, but not enough to warrant an abdominoplasty. She receives a flat, smooth abdomen with a raised mons pubis. Her smaller breasts with raised nipples are no longer ptotic.

improvement in core strength and shape (**Fig. 2**). Abdominal etching can also be created naturally through muscular development.

Through the use of electromagnetic external pulses including 6 treatments of 30 minutes per treatment over 3 weeks duration, the electromagnetic external pulsations has resulted in stronger and more toned abdominal and gluteal muscularity in both young patients and postabdominoplasty patients with 85% satisfaction (see **Fig. 1**). Should patients be dissatisfied with the technique, we provide a 50% credit of their cost to other Medi

Spa services or plastic surgery. EmSculpt has recently also been approved by the US Food and Drug Administration for extremity muscles.

PREOPERATIVE RAPID WEIGHT LOSS HUMAN CHORIOGONADOTROPIN 500 CALORIES A DAY 6-WEEK DIET

Overweight and obese individuals, especially those with excessive abdominal girth, requesting abdominoplasty are at risk for delayed wound healing and poor aesthetic results. Rather than

Fig. 5. Combining VASERlipo with BodyTite for a minimally invasive abdominoplasty in a 54-year-old woman. (*A*) Before presenting condition with presurgical markings for VASERlipo and BodyTite of anterior abdominal wall and (*B*) Four months after frontal images. (*C*) Before presenting condition with presurgical markings and (*B*) Four months after right lateral images. She has a "gap" deformity that has annoying adipose laden skin laxity, but not enough to warrant an abdominoplasty. She has a flat, smooth abdomen with naturally appearing muscular etching.

rejecting these patients, for the past 14 years our center has offered the HCG 500 calories per day diet. This diet consists of a high-protein diet and HCG injections for 6 weeks.[1,2] The HCG hormone encourages visceral fat metabolism and reduces hunger for loss of nearly a pound a day. Preoperatively treating hundreds of patients, more than 80% have lost enough weight to successfully proceed with extensive body contouring operations. The demonstrative patient is a 32-year-old woman who lost 30 pounds on the HGC program to lower her body mass index from 32 to 27 (**Fig. 3**). Her lipoabdominoplasty included imbrication of her diastasis recti and umbilical herniorrhaphy, plus VASERlipo of the flanks and lipoaugmentation of her breasts. Two years later, she has gained only 5 pounds and maintained her figure (see **Fig. 3**).

BIPOLAR RADIOFREQUENCY (BodyTite, MORPHEUS8)

Radiofrequency devices offer patients with mild skin laxity a minimally invasive option. It also expands the patient population by allowing the plastic surgeon to treat those with mild laxity who either will not consider surgery or whose deformity is as of yet too mild for surgical correction. BodyTite bipolar radiofrequency tightening offers this technology. After entry through a 14-gauge needle stick, a blunt 3-mm probe on a scissor-like bipolar handpiece emits a steady stream of energy directed to the disc receiving electrode in contact with the skin surface (Video 1). The probe is passed forward and the energy is applied on the slow back stroke for multiple passes until predetermined external and internal temperature limits are achieved. Preset temperature high limit cutoffs prevent overheating. Care in proper tissue level placement prevents burns. The end points are observable skin shrinkage, achieving designated high temperature levels, and predetermined levels of kilojoules per area. Liquefied fat is then evacuated by gentle liposuction. Incompletely damaged collagenous supporting connective tissue heals in a shortened and rejuvenated state. When properly performed, min-

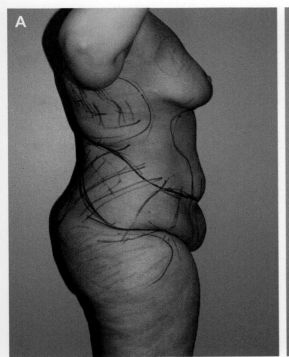
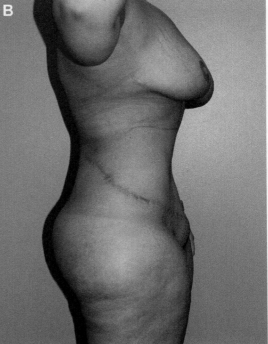

Fig. 7. Combining OFLA with strategic VASERlipo of the lateral chest, lower back with lipoaugmentation of the breasts and lateral gluteal areas to achieve an incredibly narrow and tight skin waist in a 28-year-old overweight woman, who desired to be as curvaceous as possible. (*A*) Before presenting condition with surgical markings for OFLA and VASERlipo and lipoaugmentation and (*B*) 5 months after right lateral views. Her early OLFA scars are fading within a smoothly transitioned and broadly narrowed waist. VASERlipo, which included the Flankplasty donor site and undermining neighboring areas, provided 1200 mL of processed fat for her lateral buttocks and breasts.

imal scar tissue develops, which allows for repeat BodyTite treatments to incrementally tighten tissues. Patients are informed at the outset that a second treatment may be needed for optimal skin tightening.

Sun-damaged, severely aged, and wrinkled skin may become more wrinkled after BodyTite. The immediate application of Morpheus8, a coated tip radiofrequency enhanced percutaneous microneedling, smooths out the skin. Morpheus8 has a comfortable pistol grip handpiece with 24 retractable pins that penetrate 2 to 4 mm below the skin surface to damage deep and subdermal collagen (Video 2). Over the next several months of healing, the retracted skin is less wrinkled. InMode has termed the combination of BodyTite and Morpheus8 Embrace.

The next patient demonstrates the synergism of VASERlipo and BodyTite in a 54-year-old woman who requests a flatter abdomen, narrower waist, and elimination of saddlebags (**Fig. 4**). While accepting the scars for her breast

reduction to treat symptomatic macromastia, she refused an abdominoplasty owing to pain, down time, and lengthy scar. While 1 surgical team performed her breast reduction, a second team performed VASERlipo of her abdomen, medial thighs, and saddlebags followed by Body-Tite of abdomen, medial thighs, and saddlebags. VASERlipo of her flanks did not require a change to prone position because a large gel roll was placed under her midline back. With adequate rotation of the operating room table, abdominal viscera descends away from the liposuction with each flank could be fully visualized and palpated for smooth evacuation of excess adipose. These tightly packed flanks did not need BodyTite. The complex procedure was performed in less than 2 hours as an outpatient under laryngeal mask anesthesia.

The next patient is a 49-year-old woman with a history of 2 pregnancies who desires correction of her oversized and sagging abdomen. She refused abdominoplasty and elected to undergo VASER-lipo with BodyTite and Morpheus8. After 500 mL

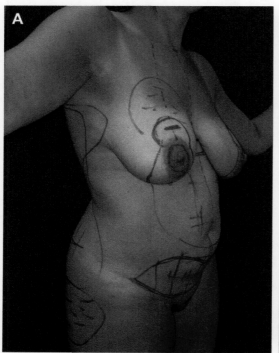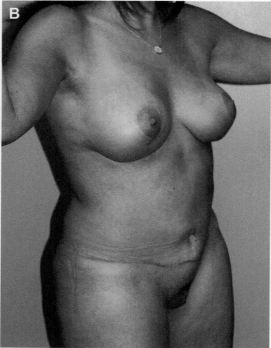

Fig. 8. Combining VASERlipo with BodyTite of the epigastrium and lateral torso with a limited abdominoplasty in a 36-year-old mother with a depressed C-section scar, and VASERlipo of her flanks and fat grafting of her lateral buttocks and superior poles of the breasts. (*A*) Before presenting condition with presurgical markings for the mastopexies, limited abdominoplasty and VASERlipo and BodyTite of anterior abdominal wall and VASERlipo of her flanks and (*B*) 6 months after right anterior oblique images. Her epigastrium is not loose enough to complete a full abdominoplasty with a low-lying scar, but loose enough to need BodyTite. She receives a flat, smooth abdomen to her mons pubis. Her smaller breasts with raised nipples are no longer ptotic. Her lateral breast roll was removed.

of tumescent (saline, xylocaine, and epinephrine) was infused into the subcutaneous tissue of her abdomen, a 3-ring VASER probe was applied at 90% for 4 minutes and 30 seconds. Then Body-Tite was applied for a total of 24 kJ with subsequent evacuation of 300 mL of emulsion through liposuction. Finally, 2 passes of Morpheus8 was performed to reduce dermal laxity and stria. Her early postoperative swelling was reduced by weekly Hyvamat electrophysiologic and VASER-shape ultrasonic lymphatic massage. **Fig. 5** shows her result at 3 months with additional contraction expected with time.

A younger patient with sagging skin and a ptotic mons pubis also declined a lipoabdomino-plasty at the time of her implant exchange with mastopexy. Instead, she underwent VASERlipo of the abdomen followed by BodyTite that extended across the mons pubis (**Fig. 6**). Four months after the procedure, she has a reduced and well-contoured abdomen and mons pubis.

VASERlipo OF REGIONS NEIGHBORING OBLIQUE FLANKPLASTY AND LIPOABDOMINOPLASTY

Strategic VASERlipo evacuation of adipose from the lateral chest, middle and low back, and epigastrium extends the reach of OFLA to reshape the entire torso. For mild to moderate localized fat deposits, VASERlipo evacuates the fat and undermines the tissues (**Fig. 7**, see Video 1). Because OFLA disrupts all but the posterior spine adherences of the torso, closure of the flank and abdomen allows circumferential skin tightening to reveal desirable body contours. Aspirated adipose is filtered to lipoaugment her buttocks and breasts as needed.

EXTENDING THE IMPACT OF A MINIABDOMINOPLASTY

Indicated for abdomens with predominantly infraumbilical excess, limited abdominoplasty without an umbilicoplasty may nevertheless leave behind epigastric laxity. BodyTite corrects the residual epigastric skin laxity to leave an overall tight result (**Fig. 8**).

SUMMARY

Candidates for abdominoplasty present a wide variety of complaints and deformities. Through searches of the Internet and the experience of friends, most patients are aware of many noninvasive and minimally invasive alternatives to open surgery. Moreover, increasing numbers are presenting with minimal deformity amenable to the limited capabilities of energy delivered alteration of tissues.

Our presentation selects a wide range of clinical scenarios for independent and complimentary use of ultrasonic assisted lipoplasty and both topical and subcutaneous use of bipolar radiofrequency tissue tightening. When adipose bulk needs to be removed, we prefer pre aspiration application of VASER ultrasonic energy to dislodge the fat, followed by BodyTite and then traditional liposuction. Because BodyTite functions best when the connective tissue is naturally stretched to length by the fat cells, we do not perform a thorough aspiration of fat before application. When there is little to no adipose excess or VASER is unavailable, preliminary liposuction is not performed.

Tissue response to properly applied radiofrequency energy is not entirely predictable. Furthermore, patients may have unrealistic expectations of result. Plastic surgeons are responsible to contrast radiofrequency tightening with the effect of more costly traditional excisional surgery. A secondary radiofrequency procedure 6 months later can have an additive effect and is easily executed owing to the limited amount of scarring from the initial procedure. Simply informing patients of the possible need for a secondary Body-Tite application emphasizes the uncertainty of results. The secondary procedural cost should be about one-half the charge for the original treatment. This offer further grounds the patient and is economically reasonable. In our practice, secondary BodyTite has been performed in approximately 25% of patients.

As an isolated procedure, BodyTite of 1 or 2 regions is performed in our office operating room under super wet local anesthesia and mild oral sedation. When BodyTite compliments major excisional body contouring, it is performed in the operating room in conjunction with the invasive operation.

The availability and use of VASER and bipolar radiofrequency provide a broad menu of options for the consumer, savvy patient and the artistic plastic surgeon. Despite the high cost of acquisition, this expanded offering is a definite practice enhancement.

DISCLOSURE

Dr D.J. Hurwitz was a paid investigator for InMode from 2010 to 2013, and has unexercised stock options. He has accepted $5000 in fees for lectures. He has received no editing or direct financial support for this article.

SUPPLEMENTARY DATA

Supplementary data related to this article can be found online at https://doi.org/10.1016/j.cps.2020.03.005.

REFERENCES

1. Hurwitz DJ, Wooten A. Plastic surgery for the obese. Int J Adipose Tis 2007;1:05–11.
2. Hurwitz DJ. In: Comprehensive body contouring: theory and practice. New York: Springer Verlag; 2016. p. 3–4.
3. Hurwitz DJ. Ultrasonic-assisted liposuction in the massive weight loss patient, Chapter 12. In: Garcia O Jr, editor. Ultrasonic lipoplasty current concepts and techniques. New York: Springer Nature; 2020. p. 189–202.
4. Hurwitz DJ. Comprehensive body contouring: theory and practice. New York: Springer Verlag; 2016. p. 12.
5. Theodorou SJ, Del Vecchio D, Chia CT. Soft tissue contraction in body contouring with radiofrequency-assisted liposuction: a treatment gap solution. Aesth Surg J 2018;38(S2):S74–8.
6. Website. Morhpeus8 clinical experience. Available at: http://www.Inmoderesources.com. Accessed October 14, 2019.
7. Hurwitz DJ, Beidas O, Wright L. Reshaping the oversized waist through Oblique Flankplasty with lipoabdominoplasty (OFLA). Plast Reconstr Surg 2019;5:960–72.
8. Clavijo-Alvarez JA, Hurwitz DJ. J torsoplasty: a novel approach to avoid circumferential scars of the upper body lift. Plast Reconstr Surg 2012;130:382e–3e.
9. Kinney BM, Lozanova P. High Intensity Electromagnetic Therapy (HIFEM) evaluated by magnetic resonance imaging (MRI): safety and efficacy of a dual tissue effect based on non-invasive abdominal wall shaping. Lasers Surg Med 2019;51(1):40–6.

Abdominoplasty After Massive Weight Loss

Jonathan P. Brower, MD[a], J. Peter Rubin, MD[b],*

KEYWORDS

- Fleur-de-lis • Vertical abdominoplasty • Body contouring • Massive weight loss • Monsplasty

KEY POINTS

- A careful evaluation of body mass index and medical comorbidities relevant to patients with massive weight loss (MWL) is essential.
- Careful analysis of the anatomic deformities in the abdominal/trunk region guides the choice of procedures to maximize patient satisfaction and avoid complications.
- The fleur-de-lis abdominoplasty is a useful operation in patients with MWL and is offered whenever there is significant horizontal skin laxity. If a patient is unsure about this option, it is always possible to perform a procedure with a transverse-only incision and selectively add in the vertical resection in a subsequent stage.
- Attention to mons ptosis, as well as excessive pubic fullness, leads to favorable outcomes. Deformity of the pubic region is often neglected in patients with MWL, but correction of the mons should be incorporated with the abdominoplasty technique.

INTRODUCTION

For patients with massive weight loss (MWL) presenting for plastic surgery consultation, the evaluation should start with the weight loss history. This conversation begins by gaining an understanding of the mechanism of weight loss, which could involve diet and exercise, sometimes supplemented with pharmacologic agents to induce weight loss, or weight loss surgery. If weight loss surgery has been performed, the type of procedure should be documented, and the plastic surgeon should classify the weight loss procedure as malabsorptive or simply restrictive. The most common malabsorptive procedure is the Roux-en-Y gastric bypass. Restrictive procedures may include vertical gastroplasty or lap band. The patient's starting weight before embarking on the weight loss journey should be documented, as well the patient's current weight and body mass index (BMI). The time course of the weight loss should also be noted. If the patient is actively losing weight, generally denoted by weight loss of more than 2.3 kg (5 pounds) a month over the preceding 3 months, surgery should be delayed until the patient has reached a plateau. Any patient who has had weight loss surgery should be queried about symptoms of dumping and nausea/vomiting. These findings are both indications that malnutrition (protein and/or micronutrient deficiency) may be present. Patients generally plateau between 12 and 18 months after weight loss surgery.[1–3]

The question of screening patients by BMI thresholds always arises. The authors use the following general framework for screening. If a patient has a BMI of 40 or more, the indications for operation should be very compelling, including a disabling giant pannus and/or severe recurrent soft tissue sepsis requiring antibiotic treatment.

[a] Department of Plastic Surgery, University of Pittsburgh Medical Center, 3380 Boulevard of the Allies, Suite 158, Pittsburgh, PA 15213, USA; [b] Department of Plastic Surgery, University of Pittsburgh Medical Center, Scaife Hall, Suite 6B, Room 690, 3550 Terrace Street, Pittsburgh, PA 15261, USA
* Corresponding author.
E-mail address: rubinjp@upmc.edu

Clin Plastic Surg 47 (2020) 389–396
https://doi.org/10.1016/j.cps.2020.03.006
0094-1298/20/© 2020 Elsevier Inc. All rights reserved.

Chronic open wounds can be another indication for operation. Otherwise, BMI should be optimized with assistance from a nutritional counseling team and the patient's bariatric surgeon, if applicable. If a patient has a BMI between 35 and 40, similar strict criteria should be applied, and the patient should be encouraged to embark on further weight loss before surgery is strongly considered. Patients presenting with a BMI of 30 to 35 are in a watershed area in which it is important to consider their overall body habitus and fat distribution in the truncal region. The most important factor is intra-abdominal adipose burden, which makes it difficult to obtain a reasonable contour on the abdomen. In contrast, patients with a BMI between 30 and 35 who have more of a gynoid body shape, with a waist-to-hip ratio of less than 1, are more suitable candidates. For patients with a BMI of 30 to 35, with significant intra-abdominal adipose tissue, further weight loss is encouraged. Patients presenting with a BMI of 25 to 30 are generally good candidates for abdominoplasty after weight loss. Some of the overall body weight is an overhanging pannus, which will be removed during surgery. Although patients with a BMI less than 25 are exceptional success stories after bariatric surgery, this end point is uncommon. When BMI is very low (eg, in the range of 20 or 21), suspicion for malnutrition should be high. It is important to keep in mind that many patients presenting for body contouring after weight loss do not have an optimized BMI and it is common to defer surgery while further weight loss is pursued[4] (**Table 1**).

Other medical comorbidities associated with obesity should be considered, including diabetes, hypertension, obstructive sleep apnea, severe arthritis, and cardiovascular disease. Presence of these morbidities may prompt further preoperative evaluation by medical consultants, as indicated. It is our practice to require patients cease use of tobacco and nicotine products at least 6 weeks before surgery.

The anatomic evaluation is very important and dictates the choice of procedure and surgical plan. Abdominal wall laxity should be assessed, as well as intra-abdominal adipose tissue mass. Prior scars should be noted. The amount of overhang of the pannus should be evaluated and the tissues under the fold of the pannus inspected for signs of chronic irritation and intertrigo. The mons region should be inspected for evidence of ptosis and excessive fullness. As an examination maneuver, the mons can be elevated manually during the examination with the patient in a standing position, to assess how much surgical elevation will be required. Importantly, the degree of horizontal laxity in the midabdomen and epigastrium should be assessed as patients are considered for a fleur-de-lis abdominoplasty. First described in 1967 by Castanares and Goethel,[5] and later popularized by Dellon,[6] the fleur-de-lis procedure should be considered in 3 circumstances: (1) excessive laxity of the epigastrium that will not be adequately corrected by inferior transposition alone; (2) presence of a prominent subcostal scar, because undermining the scar will threaten the blood supply to the inferior tissues; and (3) an assessment that a highly aggressive plication of the abdominal wall fascia is required.[7,8] Patients with extensive protrusion of the abdominal wall fascia may manifest excess skin in the epigastrium after plication, as the skin drapes unevenly over the new smaller contour of the torso. This finding should be discussed with the patient preoperatively so the patient can be involved in the decision-making process to add a vertical scar to the abdomen if necessary. The abdomen should also be assessed for a high double roll. A double roll on the midabdomen is usually easily removed with the abdominoplasty and unfurling of the abdominal flap. However, a high double roll that is just under the inframammary fold is much more difficult to eliminate with a traditional abdominoplasty approach. Additional inspection of the lateral flanks for excess adipose tissue that may be amenable to liposuction should

Table 1	
Summary of guidelines for surgical decision making based on body mass index	
BMI (kg/m²)	**Surgical Considerations**
<25	Generally excellent surgical candidates; consider nutritional deficiencies for extremely low BMI after bariatric surgery
25–30	Generally excellent surgical candidates
30–35	Surgery is considered if intra-abdominal fat burden/body habitus lend themselves to satisfactory results
35–40	Surgery is typically deferred until more weight loss is achieved; limited aesthetic results and higher risk of complications
>40	Surgery should only be considered in cases of severe functional impairment

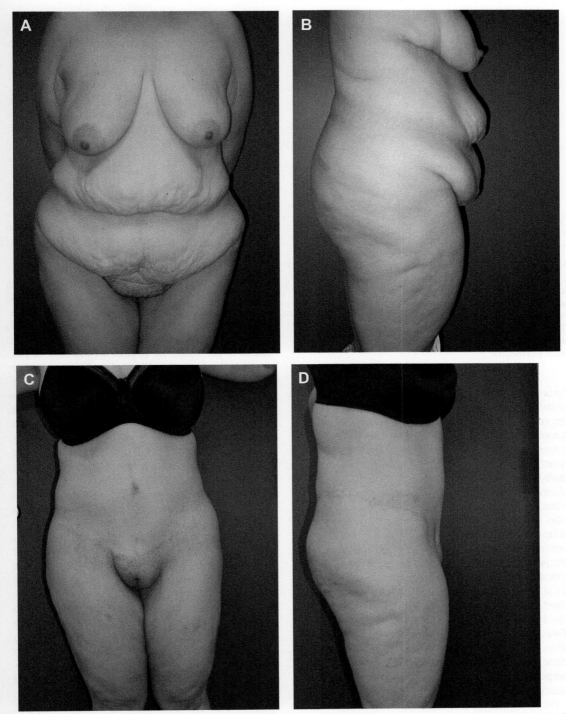

Fig. 1. A 34-year-old woman (*A, B*) before undergoing fleur-de-lis abdominoplasty and lower body lift. (*C, D*) Five-year postoperative views showing improved contour of the abdomen and mons, with enhanced shape of the waist.

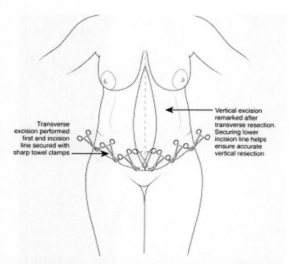

Vertical excision remarked after transverse resection. Securing lower incision line helps ensure accurate vertical resection

Transverse excision performed first and incision line secured with sharp towel clamps

Fig. 2. The transverse resection is performed first and closed temporarily with penetrating towel clips. The location of the T junction is identified. With this lower abdominal incision secured, a pinch test is used to finalize the markings for the vertical component. (*From* Mitchell RTM, Rubin JP. The Fleur-De-Lis Abdominoplasty. *Clin Plastic Surg.* 2014;41(4):673-680; with permission.)

be undertaken. In addition, the extent of circumferential skin laxity should be examined, and, as appropriate, a circumferential lower body lift approach discussed with the patient.[9] During discussion with the patient, it is vital to point out which areas will be corrected and, just as importantly, which areas will not be affected by the planned procedure. Patients may have expectations that the operation will correct rolls or loose skin on the lateral torso. Regions beyond the scope of the abdominoplasty should be pointed out and discussed in the context of potential staged or concurrent additional body contouring procedures. Likewise, in the discussion of the surgical plan, a shared decision-making approach is used and patients are given the option to defer the vertical component of an abdominoplasty if they are unsure about whether to accept the scar. Of course, when it is clearly indicated, the most cost-efficient approach for patients is to undergo a fleur-de-lis in a single-stage abdominoplasty (**Fig. 1**).

Preoperative laboratory studies should be ordered to assess any active medical comorbidities, as well as complete blood count, electrolytes, and albumin and prealbumin. These serum protein measures are important because there is a high incidence of protein malnutrition in patients who have undergone weight loss surgery and it is not possible to adequately screen these patients by

history alone.[1] In addition, patients with lap bands in place should consult with their bariatric surgeons before having body contouring surgery. Bariatric surgeons may elect to deflate the lap bad before the patient undergoes general anesthesia. All patients should be asked about personal and family history of venous thromboembolism, and additional work-up for thrombotic disorders should be commenced when indicated by history.

SURGICAL TECHNIQUE

Because this article is focused on abdominoplasty in patients with MWL, the surgical description focuses on 2 key techniques: the fleur-de-lis abdominoplasty, and mons suspension with selective manual thinning of the pubic region.

The markings for the fleur-de-lis abdominoplasty and correction of mons ptosis have common features. In all cases, whether or not a fleur-de-lis is being performed, the lower border of the abdominoplasty incision is marked with the patient pulling the skin of the abdomen in a cephalad direction to put maximal stretch on the skin of the lower abdomen and pubic region. This maneuver is most easily accomplished with the patient lying on a stretcher in a supine position but can be achieved with the patient standing, as long as the pannus is not too heavy. A mark is made directly superior to the labial commissure in the midline, 6 to 7 cm above the commissure. This mark is the lower border of the abdominoplasty incision and, importantly, correctly sets the proportions of the hair-bearing pubic skin on the abdominal wall. Next, the patient is turned to a right three-quarter view and the lateral edge of the pannus roll identified. The lateral margin of the transverse abdominal incision is marked just posterior to the edge of the roll. If the roll extends around the posterior trunk and a circumferential lower body lift is not planned in this operative session, then the transverse lower abdominal incision should terminate on the roll, rather than in a crease below the roll. This maneuver runs the dog-ear into a natural roll, and it creates a less noticeable feature. The patient is then turned the left three-quarter view and the opposite lateral margin of the low transverse incision is marked in a location symmetric to the right side. In some cases, patients have a natural asymmetry of the tissues that requires asymmetric placement of the lateral margins of the incisions to encompass additional tissue or adjust to the location of various skin rolls. The patient is then asked to hold up the pannus with maximal stretch on the skin of the lower abdomen and pubis once again. At this point, the

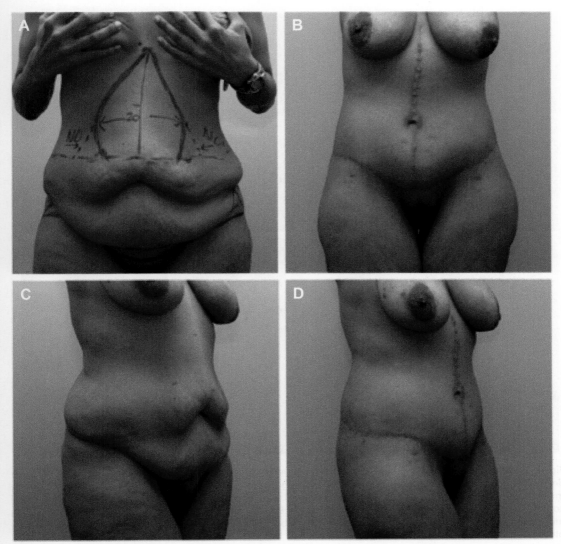

Fig. 3. A 40-year-old woman undergoing fleur-de-lis abdominoplasty. (*A, C*) Preoperative markings indicating medial bias at the caudal margin of the vertical resection. (*B, D*) Postoperative views showing improved contour of the lower abdomen and waist. (*From* Hunstad JP, Kortesis BG, Knotts CD. Fleur-de-lis abdominoplasty including mons contouring. In: Rubin JP, Jewell ML, Richter DF, Uebel CO, eds. *Body Contouring and Liposuction*. Philadelphia, PA: Elsevier; 2013: 254-264; with permission.)

lateral margins that had been marked for the low transverse incision are connected with a continuous line to the mark at the midline. The low transverse incision that has been marked may appear to be below the inguinal ligament when the tissues are relaxed. However, note that the scar will ultimately end up in its position when the patient had the tissue on stretch. The extent of the vertical resection is estimated with a pinch test, with final markings confirmed on the operating table. The pitfall of any pinch test maneuver is that it fails to

accurately account for the thickness of the double layer of subcutaneous tissue between the fingers.

Following induction of general anesthesia with sequential compression devices (SCDs) in place and activated, the patient is positioned supine on the operating table. A dilute epinephrine solution (1 mg of 1:1000 epinephrine in 100 mL of saline) is infiltrated intradermally along the lower abdominal incision. Medially, the incision is carried directly down to the muscle fascia. Laterally, dissection is carried cephalad, particularly in those

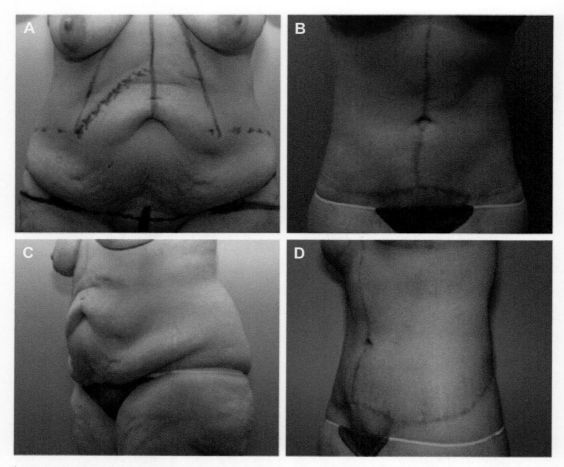

Fig. 4. A 50-year-old woman with a history of massive weight loss and open cholecystectomy undergoing fleur-de-lis abdominoplasty. (*A, C*) Preoperative views showing markings, including the right upper quadrant abdominal scar to be included within the vertical resection. (*B, D*) Postoperative views showing improved abdominal contour and waist shape. (*From* Hunstad JP, Kortesis BG, Knotts CD. Fleur-de-lis abdominoplasty including mons contouring. In: Rubin JP, Jewell ML, Richter DF, Uebel CO, eds. Body Contouring and Liposuction. Philadelphia, PA: Elsevier; 2013: 254-264; with permission.)

patients with MWL in whom the lower abdominal marking is below the inguinal ligament. In this scenario, the dissection proceeds down to the muscle fascia only once it has crossed the level of the inguinal ligament. The flap is elevated centrally along the muscle fascia, with just enough lateral dissection to permit natural redraping of the abdominal flap. Extensive lateral undermining increases surgical dead space without providing aesthetic benefit and threatens the blood supply to the lower abdominal flaps. A key tenet of this procedure is to avoid extensive undermining and make every effort to preserve perforating vessels above the umbilicus. The surgeon should conceptualize that, in the region above the umbilicus, undermining is performed only beneath the area of planned resection.

The amount of fat left adherent to the abdominal wall is at the surgeon's discretion but should be informed by any plan to plicate the rectus sheath. The umbilicus is dissected from the abdominal flap, ensuring the stalk is not denuded of sufficient adherent fat for optimal perfusion. The operating table is then flexed to determine extent of resection relative to the aesthetic result and tension of closure. At this point, the T-junction location is estimated. A penetrating towel clip is secured to the lower wound edge and gently transposed cephalad. The towel clip is palpated through the upper abdominal flap and marked. A line connecting these markings with the planned corners safely and reliably demarcates the superior extent of the resection. The planned abdominal flap excision is then completed, keeping the subcutaneous tissue

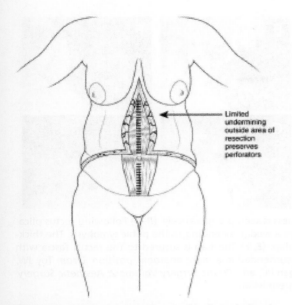

Limited
undermining
outside area of
resection
preserves
perforators

Fig. 5. Final resection pattern in the fleur-de-lis abdominoplasty. Undermining of the abdominal flap is limited to the area to be resected to preserve perforating vessels and optimize perfusion of the caudal flap. (*From* Mitchell RTM, Rubin JP. The Fleur-De-Lis Abdominoplasty. Clin Plastic Surg. 2014;41(4):673-680; with permission.)

flush with the skin edge to ensure a smooth contour across the incision closure. If a fleur-de-lis procedure is planned, this transverse abdominal excision is completed before proceeding with the vertical component of the procedure. This lower abdominal incision is approximated and secured with towel clips to prevent distraction during the vertical resection (**Fig. 2**).

If vertical resection is planned, it is double checked on the table with another pinch test beginning just caudal to the xiphoid, extending to the inferior margin of the abdominal flap. Importantly, the marking is adjusted at this caudal-most point such that the markings are biased more medially (**Fig. 3**). This maneuver conserves more skin at the T junction to minimize tension at this critical point. The technique affords the surgeon the discretion to adjust these markings to account for asymmetric adiposity and abdominal scars to optimize contour and minimize tissue ischemia (**Fig. 4**). These markings are then infiltrated with epinephrine solution before excision is undertaken. Dissection proceeds directly down to rectus fascia, carefully avoiding undermining of the abdominal flaps, which would increase the risk of wound complications (**Fig. 5**). Judicious debulking is often necessary at the most superior

portion of the incision to improve contour and avoid a dog-ear.[10]

Before incisions are closed, the mons is evaluated for excess laxity and thickness relative to the abdominal flap. These findings are addressed by debulking the area with direct fat excision and securing it to the underlying muscle fascia with permanent braided suture[11,12] (**Fig. 6**).

Tailor tacking begins at the T junction, ensuring the desired contour is achieved and excessive tension is avoided. The incisions are closed over 2 or 3 drains, beginning with the superficial fascial system (SFS) within the limits of the hair-bearing pubic region only. Deep sutures lateral to this landmark may be palpable and do not significantly reduce the tension of closure. The vertical incision is closed beginning with deep sutures in the SFS. To avoid widening and distortion of the umbilicus, it is inset within the vertical incision without any additional skin excision of the abdominal flap. A running intradermal barbed suture is used to close the skin before it is dressed with skin glue.

POSTOPERATIVE MANAGEMENT AND COMPLICATIONS

The patient is immediately placed in an abdominal binder and transferred to a hospital bed, maintaining flexion at the hips during transfer. Overnight observation is encouraged to promote early ambulation and monitor for signs of bleeding. SCDs are maintained while the patient is admitted, especially before ambulation. Drains are removed when output decreases to less than 30 mL in a 24-hour period. Once drains have been removed, the binder may be replaced with a compression garment for a total of 6 weeks. Vigorous physical activity and heavy lifting are minimized during this period, although frequent ambulation is encouraged.[13]

Complication rates for abdominoplasty vary in the literature, but are up to twice as high among patients with MWL. Wound complications are the most common, particularly in the fleur-de-lis abdominoplasty, likely as a result of compromised perfusion at the T junction. These wound complications are typically limited to dehiscence, infection, and minor skin necrosis; major skin loss requiring reoperation is unusual. Seroma rates vary in the literature but are reportedly as high as 22%. Most seromas are managed conservatively in the office with serial aspiration or drain replacement, but some require surgical excision of the cavity. These revisions may be incorporated into planned future body contouring procedures. Current literature suggests there is not a significant difference in seroma and hematoma

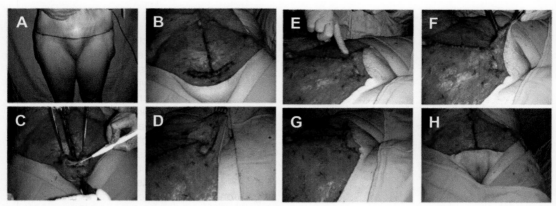

Fig. 6. Mons debulking and resuspension. (*A*) Mons fullness is seen preoperatively. (*B–D*) Following rectus plication, the planned mons resection is marked and excised as a wedge extending to the pubic symphysis. The thickness of the mons should match that of the abdominal flap. (*E, F*) The flap is secured to the rectus fascia with braided permanent sutures. (*G, H*) The debulked flap is suspended in a more anatomic position. (*From* Toy JW, Rubin JP. Post-bariatric reconstruction. In: Rubin JP, Neligan PC, eds. *Plastic Surgery Volume 2: Aesthetic Surgery.* 4th ed. Philadelphia, PA: Elsevier; 2018:709-730.e3; with permission.)

rates between traditional and fleur-de-lis abdominoplasty.[11]

SUMMARY

Fleur-de-lis abdominoplasty is a powerful technique to shape the abdomen and waist in patients with MWL, and it may be combined with a lower body lift for circumferential contouring of the torso. Deformity of the mons can be reliably addressed concurrently. Although it is most cost-effective to simultaneously address vertical and horizontal laxity simultaneously, the vertical component of the operation can be deferred safely if the patient is not prepared to accept an obvious abdominal scar. Strict criteria for patient selection should be applied, particularly with respect to BMI and medical comorbidities.

DISCLOSURE

The authors have nothing to disclose.

REFERENCES

1. Naghshineh N, Coon DO, McTigue K, et al. Nutritional assessment of bariatric surgery patients presenting for plastic surgery: a prospective analysis. Plast Reconstr Surg 2010;126:602–10.

2. Bossert RP, Rubin JP. Evaluation of the weight loss patient presenting for plastic surgery consultation. Plast Reconstr Surg 2012;130:1361–9.

3. Michael J, Coon D, Rubin JP. Complications in postbariatric body contouring: strategies for assessment and prevention. Plast Reconstr Surg 2011;127:1352–7.

4. Coon D, Gusenoff JA, Kannan N, et al. Body mass and surgical complications in the postbariatric reconstructive patient: analysis of 511 cases. Ann Surg 2009;249:397–401.

5. Castanares S, Goethel JA. Abdominal lipectomy: a modification in technique. Plast Reconstr Surg 1967;40:378–83.

6. Dellon AL. Fleur-de-lis abdominoplasty. Aesthet Plast Surg 1985;9:27–32.

7. Friedman T, Wiser I. Abdominal contouring and combining procedures. Clin Plast Surg 2019;46:41–8.

8. Hunstad JP, Kortesis BG, Knotts CD. Fleur-de-lis abdominoplasty including mons contouring. In: Rubin JP, Jewell ML, Richter DF, editors. Body contouring and liposuction. New York: Elsevier; 2013. p. 254–64.

9. Toy JW, Rubin JP. Post-bariatric reconstruction. In: Rubin JP, Neligan PC, et al, editors. Plastic surgery. New York: Elsevier; 2018. p. 709–30.

10. Mitchell RTM, Rubin JP. The Fleur-De-Lis abdominoplasty. Clin Plast Surg 2014;41:673–80.

11. Friedman T, Coon DO, Michaels J, et al. Fleur-de-Lis abdominoplasty: a safe alternative to traditional abdominoplasty for the massive weight loss patient. Plast Reconstr Surg 2010;125:1525–35.

12. Bykowski MR, Rubin JP, Gusenoff JA. The impact of abdominal contouring with monsplasty on sexual function and urogenital distress in women following massive weight loss. Aesthet Surg J 2017;37:63–70.

13. Wallach SG. Abdominal contour surgery for the massive weight loss patient: the Fleur-De-Lis approach. Aesthet Surg J 2005;25:454–65.

Abdominal Etching

Ahmad Saad, MD[a],*, Luciano Nahas Combina, MD[b,1],
Carlos Altamirano-Arcos, MD[b,2]

KEYWORDS

- High-definition liposculpture • Body contouring • Power-assisted liposuction • Lipoplasty

KEY POINTS

- Mentz first described the abdominal etching technique in the 1990s. It has gained popularity over the last 10 years with the development of new technologies and the growing ability of plastic surgeons to precisely sculpt the abdominal wall.
- Reciprocating power-assisted liposuction permits the complete evacuation of the deep fat compartment and allows for safe and precise sculpture of anatomic landmarks following the underlying muscular-skeletal frame.
- The extent of abdominal etching is offered in low, medium, or high grade of definition, and it is controlled by the surgeon depending on the amount of superficial liposuction and fat redistribution.
- Long-term results are maintained over time with the proper nutritional and exercising routine.

INTRODUCTION

Liposuction has become a popular procedure since the early 1980s. According to the 2018 report from the American Society for Aesthetic Plastic Surgery, the second most popular cosmetic procedure was liposuction, with more than 280,000 procedures in the United States.[1]

Over the last 30 years, liposuction technologies have evolved, and new techniques for abdominal etching have been described. These technologies fall under five major families based on their mechanism of action: (1) suction-assisted liposuction, (2) ultrasound-assisted liposuction, (3) laser-assisted liposuction, (4) power-assisted liposuction (PAL), and (5) radiofrequency-based lipectomy.[2,3] This technological advancement permitted liposuction to be performed with fewer complication rates while improving patient safety and achieving better aesthetic results.[4] These improvements have contributed to the positioning of liposuction as one of the most popular aesthetic procedures and have made it a more attractive option for patients seeking to improve their physical appearance, contour their figure, and achieve results that cannot be obtained solely with diet and exercise.

Abdominal etching is a group of techniques described to improve the aesthetics of the abdominal region using liposuction and fat redistribution; nevertheless, the abdominal unit cannot be aesthetically separated from the rest of the torso. Therefore, the authors recommend the treatment of the chest, abdomen, and lower back simultaneously to achieve an aesthetically pleasant and harmonic appearance. The authors have found that good surgical outcomes and postoperative profiles are achieved with the use of the PAL technology for abdominal etching (**Box 1**).[5,6]

This article offers a comprehensive description of the authors' technique, including preoperative

[a] IMAGN Institute, rambla Catalunya 43 Ent 1, Barcelona 08007, Spain; [b] Hospital General "Dr. Manuel Gea González," Mexico City, Mexico
[1] Present address: Av. San Fernando 43, Col. Toriello Guerra, Del. Tlalpan, CP 14050, Ciudad de México, México.
[2] Present address: Alica 76, Col. Molino del Rey, Del. Miguel Hidalgo, CP 11040, Ciudad de México, México.
* Corresponding author.
E-mail address: ahmadsaad78@gmail.com
Twitter: @drlucianonahas (L.N.C.); @DrAltamiranoA (C.A.-A.)

Clin Plastic Surg 47 (2020) 397–408
https://doi.org/10.1016/j.cps.2020.03.001

assessment, intraoperative procedure, and postoperative care for patients undergoing abdominal etching. Other subjects discussed include historical perspective, anatomic considerations, and complications. The content of this article assists plastic surgeons in delivering consistent and predictable abdominal etching results.

HISTORICAL PERSPECTIVE

In 1977 Fisher used the term "liposuction" and described the suction-assisted lipectomy method.[7] In 1980, Illouz[8] introduced blunt instrumentation, which removed fat while minimizing trauma to the surrounding structures coursing between the undersurface of the dermis and the subjacent muscle fascia. In 1998, the US Food and Drug Administration approved PAL technology. This mechanically reciprocating technology (2000–4000 cpm) recreates the forward and backward motion of the operator's arm with the cannula tip. The low reciprocating amplitude of the cannula tip (3 mm), combined with the negative pressure, allows the surgeon to precisely sculpt the superficial fat layer in addition to suctioning the deep fat layer.[9] Under magnification, it is demonstrated how PAL is less traumatic to structures surrounding the aspirated fat.[10]

Abdominal etching was first described by Mentz and colleagues[11] in 1993 to enhance abdominal definition in bodybuilders. In 2007 Hoyos and Millard[12] described the high-definition liposculpture technique with the use of vibration amplification of sound energy at resonance, and it involves several techniques that are designed to emulate athletic and attractive surface anatomy in males and females.

ANATOMY OF THE ABDOMINAL REGION

To achieve a natural-looking and defined abdomen, it is of utmost importance to have a profound understanding of the anterior abdominal wall anatomy. Each layer of the anterior abdominal wall (muscles and muscle fascia, deep fat layer,

superficial fat layer, and skin) has to be evaluated to achieve the desired patient outcome. Abdominal contour is substantially affected by age, genetics, muscular mass, tone, obesity, parity, and posture.

Descriptive Anatomy of the Abdominal Region

The anterior abdominal wall is limited superiorly by the costal margins and the xiphoid, and inferiorly by the iliac crests, inguinal ligaments, pubic crest, and pubic symphysis. Its lateral margins are defined by vertical lines dropped from the costal margins to the most elevated portion of the iliac crests (medial axillary line).

The linea alba extends in the midline from the pubic symphysis to the xiphoid process, and it is divided by the umbilicus into the supraumbilical and infraumbilical area. The muscular wall of the anterior abdomen is composed of the external and internal oblique, transverse, rectus abdominis, and the pyramidalis muscles.

The rectus abdominal muscles consist of vertically oriented paired bellies, not necessarily symmetric, that occupies most of the central part of the anterior abdominal wall. They are separated in the midline by the linea alba and by three horizontal tendinous intersections (inscriptions). Usually, there is one pair of inscriptions at the level of the xiphoid, another around the umbilicus, and one between these two structures. There is a depression on the lateral margin of each rectus muscle that consists of the anatomic transition between the rectus muscle and the external oblique. This depression creates the linea semilunaris.[13,14] The visible shape of the anterior abdominal wall is the result of the layered osteomyofascial system, deep fat tissue, superficial fascial system, superficial fat layer, and the skin. The interactions among all these layers create the aesthetic contour through light reflection differences from prominences and shadows from depressions (**Fig. 1**).

Adipose Tissue Layers

A profound understanding of the three-dimensional anatomy of the fat layers is key to perform abdominal etching procedures.[15] Abdominal fat layers are practically divided into superficial and deep layers separated by the superficial fascia.[16]

The deep adipose tissue layer lies under the Scarpa fascia (superficial fascia) and above the muscular fascia. It is composed of large, loose, and less compact fat and can often be safely aspirated without creating any significant contour irregularities.[17]

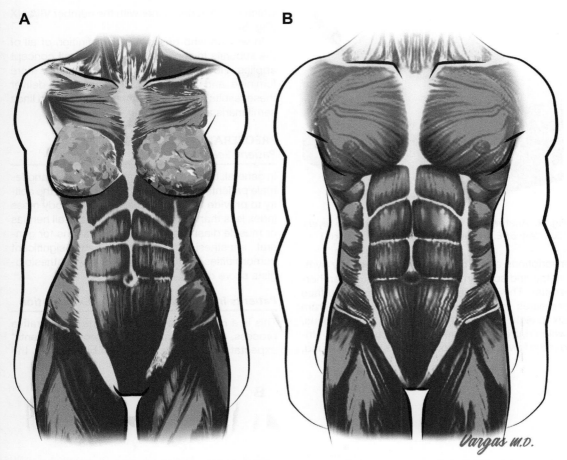

Fig. 1. The anatomy of the anterior abdominal wall. (*A*) Female anterior abdominal wall. (*B*) Male anterior abdominal wall. (*Courtesy of* E. Vargas, MD, Mexico City, Mexico.)

The superficial adipose tissue layer is located between the dermis and the superficial fascia and is composed of denser, tightly adherent fat cells. Precise sculpting for abdominal etching is achieved by performing liposuction in this superficial layer. Note that above the umbilicus, most of the fat is located in the superficial layer, whereas below the umbilicus, it is found mainly in the deep layer (**Fig. 2**).

According to the distribution of fat layers, we propose the term lipocontouring (LC) for deep fat liposuction and superficial fat liposculpting (SFLS) for superficial liposuction. It has been previously demonstrated that superficial liposuction, using proper technique, preserves the skin microvascular network of the abdominal wall.[18]

Topographic Anatomy/Abdominal Subunits

The medial abdomen (zone 1) is the area that overlies the rectus muscles bordered laterally by the linea semilunaris. The lateral abdomen (zone 2) is the territory that extends beyond linea semilunaris. This area is in continuation with the lower back posteriorly and the serratus triangle (zone 3) superiorly (**Fig. 3**).

The serratus triangle (zone 3) is the area that is bordered anteriorly by the oblique lateral edge of the pectoralis muscle, posteriorly by the latissimus dorsi, overlying the serratus muscles, and in continuation with zone 2 inferiorly (**Fig. 4**).

The term "six-packs" refers to the rectus muscle subunits. These bellies are separated vertically by the linea alba and horizontally by the abdominal inscriptions. The inscriptions are tendinous connections between the rectus muscle subunits with high anatomic variability. In general, the lower pair of inscriptions are located around the level of the umbilicus, whereas the highest couple of inscriptions are around the level of the xiphoid. Another pair of inscriptions is usually present between these two structures. Note that the

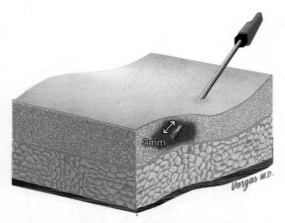

Fig. 2. Anatomy of superficial and deep fat layers. (*Courtesy of* E. Vargas, MD, Mexico City, Mexico.)

inscriptions are almost always not perfectly symmetric and sometimes are more oblique than horizontal. The external anterior abdominal surface recreates rounded square areas that vary from six to eight subunits (I to VIII) above the umbilicus, which represent the underlying rectus bellies. Under the lowest inscription, an odd subunit is found,

which is nominated either with the number VII or IX (**Fig. 5**).

In women who desire a high definition of all of the subunits in zone 1, the same subunit concept applies. However, most women request a more feminine and less defined physique. To deliver these results, delineation of the linea alba and linea semilunaris alone is enough.

PREOPERATIVE CONSIDERATIONS
Patient Selection

In general, this procedure is offered to male and female patients, older than 18 years old with the ability to provide informed consent, with a body mass index less than 30, without abdominal wall hernias or muscle diastasis, no contraindications for general anesthesia, and without any significant comorbidities (American Society of Anesthesiologists score of 2 or less).

Patients Interview and Physical Examination

This is a remarkable instance of the preoperative process, where the physician listens to patients' expectations and clears all doubts. During the

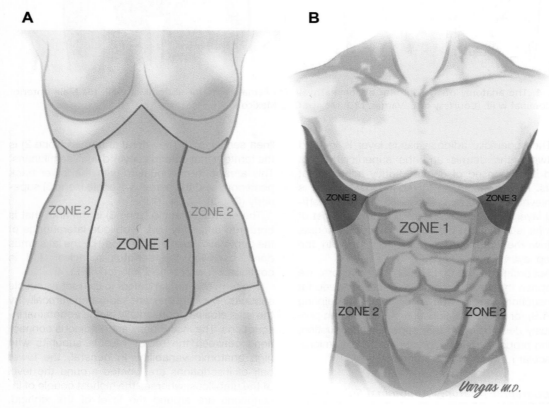

Fig. 3. Abdominal aesthetic subunits. (*A*) Female anterior subunits. (*B*) Male anterior subunits. Zone 1, medial abdomen. Zone 2, lateral abdomen. Zone 3, serratus triangle. (*Courtesy of* E. Vargas, MD, Mexico City, Mexico.)

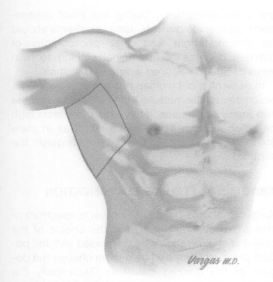

Fig. 4. Serratus triangle. (*Courtesy of* E. Vargas, MD, Mexico City, Mexico.)

initial interview, the surgeon should go over patients' age, history of pregnancy and mode of delivery, past and present medical and surgical history, allergies, and history of medication and supplements intake. During the physical

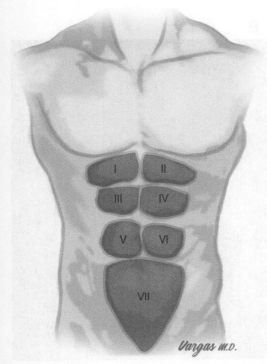

Fig. 5. "Six-pack" subunits. (*Courtesy of* E. Vargas, MD, Mexico City, Mexico.)

examination, height, weight, and body mass index need to be calculated, and key elements should be identified and discussed (**Box 2**)[19]:

In this initial consultation, the surgeon must show before and after photographs of other patients to estimate the extent of the desired definition that the patient is requesting.

Safety Selection Criteria

- Nonsmokers. Patients who smoke are encouraged to stop smoking 2 to 3 weeks before surgery until 6 weeks after the procedure.[7]
- Patients are encouraged to have a healthy lifestyle, including diet and exercise.
- Medications and supplements must be reviewed in detail.
- Absence of hernias to avoid the injury of intraabdominal structures.

Photographic Assessment

Reliable preoperative photographs are essential for clinical and scientific purposes. Photographs should be taken with the patient in a standing position to reliably assess the anatomy and be able to make a comparison with postoperative follow-up.

The patient must stay at rest without actively making any effort or contraction. Four photographic positions are required: (1) frontal view, (2) side view, (3) oblique view, and (4) posterior view.

PREOPERATIVE PLANNING AND PREPARATION
Male Abdominal Etching Marking

The marking process should follow patients' anatomic landmarks at all times. This usually demands an in-depth anatomic evaluation, and the surgeon should devote the necessary time to accurately mark the patient's anatomy. The underlying bony and muscular anatomy are the guidelines. The patient's marking is a dynamic process

---

Box 2
Physical examination key points

- Profound evaluation of skin quality (thickness and laxity)
- Superficial and deep fat layers (pinch test)
- Abdominal muscle integrity and strength (tone, volume, if they are palpable or not)
- Previous scars
- Presence of hernias

that requires a continuous contraction and relaxation of the abdominal muscles.

The Sequence of Marking

1. Midline from the sternal notch to the umbilicus and from the umbilicus to the pubic area
2. Inferior costal margin
3. Inframammary fold
4. Rectus abdominis muscle subunits, starting with the six to eight units above the umbilicus
5. Inferior rectus muscle subunit and its lateral border down to the level of the inguinal region

Once this is achieved, the linea alba and the linea semilunaris are automatically evident without the need for further marking. The superior extent of the abdominal etching should reach around the level of the lower border of the pectoralis muscle.

The key step for abdominal etching is identifying the abdominal intersections and bellies that must be palpated and precisely marked one by one respecting the underlying natural anatomy. It should be considered that sometimes bellies are not parallelly disposed and symmetric.

Female Abdominal Etching Marking

The process of abdominal etching in women follows the same initial steps as in men, but there are some exceptions. During the initial assessment, as in male patients, female patients should be shown before and after photographs of different degrees of abdominal etching to help them decide the desired extent of definition.

In general, most women request mild definition, which means the marking of the linea alba and the two lineae semilunaris. If the patient requests high definition in zone 1, the same steps as in male marking should be followed to distinguish the subunits.

ABDOMINAL ETCHING CLASSIFICATION

Surgeons should be able to deliver a spectrum of abdominal etching levels, and the choice of the extent of etching should be discussed with the patient preoperatively and help them choose the degree of the desired definition. Technically the surgeon can manage the level of definition by controlling the differential level of fat that is preserved in the superficial fat layer and the sharpness of the edges and the points of transition. We propose the following classification based on the extent of SFLS:

A. Low-definition abdominal etching (**Figs. 6–8**)
B. Medium-definition abdominal etching (**Figs. 9 and 10**)

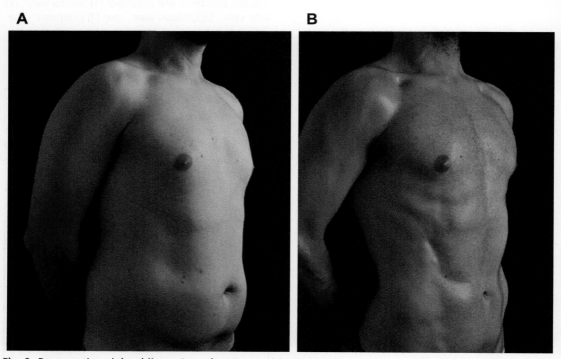

A   **B**

Fig. 6. Preoperative, right oblique view of a 32-year-old patient with a body mass index of 28.4 (*A*). Postoperative, right oblique view, after a mild-definition abdominal etching (*B*).

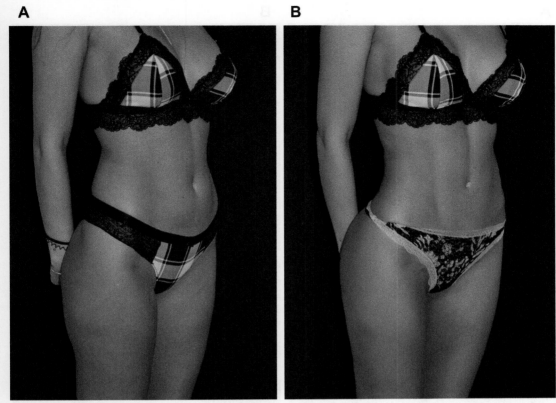

A   B

Fig. 7. Preoperative, right oblique view of a female 36-year-old patient with a body mass index of 22.5 (*A*). Postoperative, right oblique view, after a mild-definition abdominal etching (*B*).

C. High-definition abdominal etching (**Figs. 11** and **12**)

It is essential to notice that most women are included in the low-definition category.

SURGICAL TECHNIQUE

All patients undergo general anesthesia and endotracheal intubation. To monitor urine output, a urinary catheter is placed. We use intermittent pneumatic compression because it is recommended for deep vein thrombosis prophylaxis.[20,21] Supine position with extended arms is preferred. Preparation for abdominal etching begins with a chlorhexidine wash to decrease the bacterial skin load. A dressing is placed over the genitalia and arms, lower limbs, and lateral abdomen are covered with surgical drapes. All patients receive one dose of intravenous cefazolin a few minutes before incision.

Infiltration

Wetting solution (1000 mL of 0.9% NaCl, 20 mL of 1% lidocaine, 1 mL [1:1000] epinephrine) is injected through 5-mm incisions in the following sites in men: bilateral paramedian suprapubic region, intraumbilical, and within the nipple-areola complex bilaterally. In women the following sites are similarly injected: bilateral paramedian suprapubic region and intraumbilical incisions. If women desire high definition of abdominal subunits in zone 1, bilateral inframammary fold incisions are made to create the "six-packs."

Through the paramedian suprapubic incisions, we infiltrate deep fat from zone 1 and 2. Zone 3 is infiltrated through the nipple-areola complex incisions. The linea alba and the abdominal inscriptions are infiltrated through the umbilicus. To optimize the epinephrine and lidocaine effect of the wetting solution, we wait 15 minutes before moving to the next step.

Dispersion

This phase consists of the use of PAL vibratory energy while the suction power is deactivated. During this step, we treat the infiltrated areas to maximize the interaction between the tumescent fluid and the fat tissue. This should

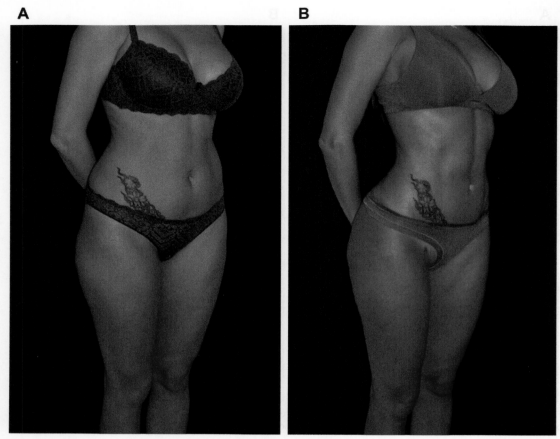

Fig. 8. Preoperative, right oblique view of a female 39-year-old patient with a body mass index of 21.8 (*A*). Postoperative, right oblique view, after a mild-definition abdominal etching (*B*).

enhance the effect of lidocaine and epinephrine in the treatment zone, decreasing the bleeding ratio, and optimizing the quality of harvested fat.

Aspiration

Liposuction is performed using the PAL system. Superficial and deep fat harvesting is done with 5-mm PAL HD cannulas (Microaire, Inc, Charlottesville, VA) (**Fig. 13**).

The process of abdominal etching is divided into two different phases. The first one is LC, which consists of the extraction of the deep fat under Scarpa fascia. Zones 1, 2, and 3 are treated until all deep fat is entirely aspirated.

The SFLS consists of the detailed sculpting of the superficial fat that allows the enhancement of the underlying musculoskeletal structures. Fat should be aspirated following the markings as guidelines at all times. The superficial fat is extracted along the linea alba, linea semilunaris,

and underlying inscriptions. There is no limit on the number of passes in the same area. It is imperative to avoid torque movements while the cannula is intracorporeal to preserve the integrity of perforator vessels and reduce ecchymosis and postoperative edema.[13]

Abdominal inscriptions overlying the rectus abdominis are marked through the umbilicus and the nipple-areola complexes without the need for additional incisions. This is accomplished with the use of the straight and curved PAL HD cannulas. We called this technique the "serpentine technique" because the cannula tip is guided through the superficial fat layer with 180° intracorporeal cannula rotations of the curved PAL HD cannula following the preoperative markings to create the inscriptions. The extent of the definition depends on the edge sharpness created in the superficial fat layer and the amount of fat that is preserved from this layer. This should be guided by the patient's desire and preoperative plan (**Box 3**).

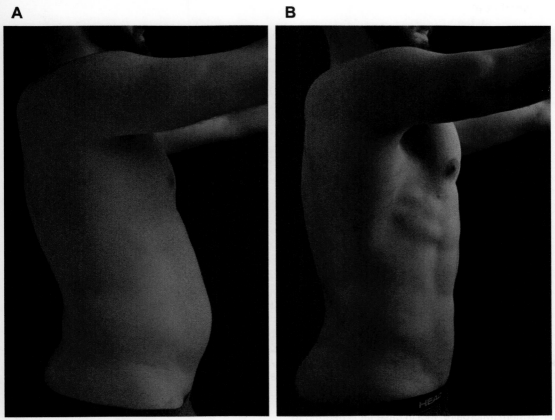

Fig. 9. Preoperative, right lateral view of a male 29-year-old patient with a body mass index of 24.2 (*A*). Postoperative, right lateral view, after a medium-definition abdominal etching (*B*).

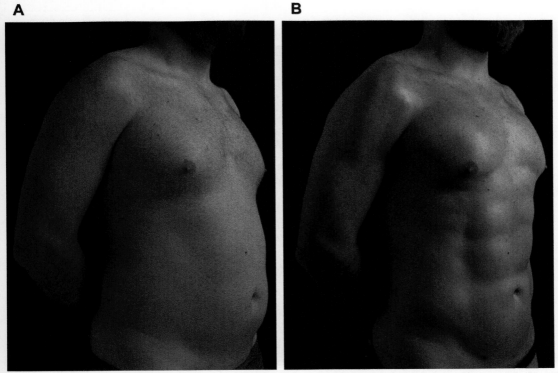

Fig. 10. Preoperative, right oblique view of a male 34-year-old patient with a BMI of 27.3 (*A*). Postoperative, right lateral view, after a medium-definition abdominal etching (*B*).

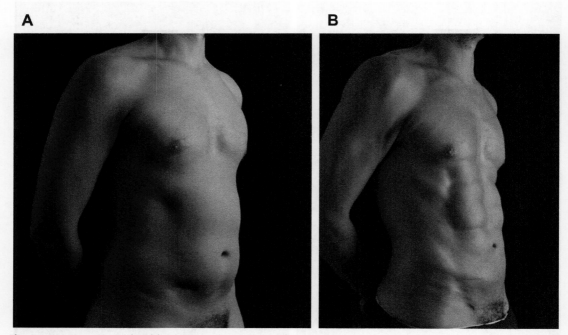

Fig. 11. Preoperative, right oblique view of a male 27-year-old patient with a BMI of 24.9 (*A*). Postoperative, right lateral view, after a high-definition abdominal etching (*B*).

Fat is collected and processed using the Lipofilter System (Microaire, Inc) in case fat is needed to graft and augment the abdominal six-packs or any other body region.

Fat Equalization

This is the final step for abdominal etching. It consists of using the reciprocating mechanical energy of the PAL technology without the need for

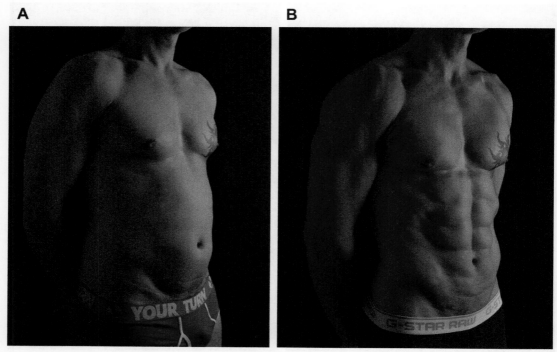

Fig. 12. Preoperative, right lateral view of a male 30-year-old patient with a BMI of 26.9 (*A*). Postoperative, right lateral view, after a high-definition abdominal etching (*B*).

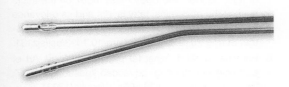

Fig. 13. MicroAire PAL HD cannulas. (*Courtesy of* Microaire, Inc, Charlottesville, VA.)

suction. This is an essential step to smoothen the superficial fat layer and correct any step-offs that were created during the process. The cannula is used to facilitate the transposition of viable fat cells into areas that need to be increased or filled.[22]

No drains are placed. A single intradermal absorbable suture is used to close the incisions, and dressings are applied. After all wounds are closed and dressings are applied, compression foam (Epi-foam, Biodermis, Inc, Henderson, NV) strips are disposed over the superficially marked areas.

POSTOPERATIVE CARE

Patients are usually discharged on Day 1 after the procedure and evaluated periodically on Day 7, Day 21, 3 months, 6 months, and 1 year. Early mobilization is encouraged to reduce the risk of thromboembolic events.

Good adjuvant therapy includes lymphatic massage, which is scheduled to start between postoperative days 5 to 7, for two sessions per 6 weeks. Manual lymphatic massage involves draining the swelling areas to the closest lymph nodes, especially in LC fat areas, to avoid fibrosis development and enhance the abdominal etching.

We usually prescribe paracetamol and ibuprofen for postoperative analgesia. Based on our previous publication, all patients were completely off pain medication within 1 week of surgery.[23]

Epifoam is removed at postoperative day 5. Compression garments are used for 3 weeks.

Box 3
Abdominal etching technique key points

- Follow the preoperative marking at all times
- No torque movement
- Use the serpentine technique to create the abdominal inscriptions through intracorporeal rotations of the curved PAL HD cannula

---

Patients may return to work after 6 days. By three weeks, they are capable of returning to full activity and standard exercise routines. We recommend avoiding water sports until every incision is healed.

The late postoperative care includes nutritional control and continuous weight control. Definitive results of abdominal etching are evaluated after 1 year. Maintaining long-term outcomes depends on dietary adherence and patient's workout regimen. Long-term outcomes and the definition grade of abdominal wall musculature acquired by etching are affected by weight gain. That is why we emphasize the importance of patient selection criteria and preoperative patient counseling.

COMPLICATIONS

Complications are divided into two groups: major and minor. Major complications are defined as an event that needs hospital readmission or new surgical intervention. Those are similar to any other liposuction procedure and include hematoma, deep vein thrombosis, pulmonary embolism, fat embolism, and abdominal wall perforation. Such major complications are rare. Minor complications are the most frequent and include: contour irregularities, reduced level of definition, fluid collections, and wound healing alterations.

Fluid collections are drained under local anesthesia. Contour irregularities are usually caused by fibrosis between the skin and underlying fascia and is treated by acoustic shock wave therapy. If excessive fibrosis develops, combining transcutaneous ultrasound with manual massage can help to solve this issue.

DISCLOSURE

Dr A. Saad is a consultant for Microaire.

REFERENCES

1. Available at: https://www.surgery.org/sites/default/files/ASAPS-Stats2018_0.pdf. Accessed September 28, 2019.
2. Tabbal GN, Ahmad J, Lista F, et al. Advances in liposuction: five key principles with emphasis on patient safety and outcomes. Plast Reconstr Surg Glob Open 2013;1(8):e75.
3. Berry MG, Davies D. Liposuction: a review of principles and techniques. J Plast Reconstr Aesthet Surg 2011;64(8):985–92.
4. Ahmad J, Eaves FF, Rohrich RJ, et al. The American Society for Aesthetic Plastic Surgery (ASAPS) survey: current trends in liposuction. Aesthet Surg J 2011;31(2):214–24.
5. Saad AN, Arbelaez JP, de Benito J. High definition liposculpture in male patients using reciprocating

power-assisted liposuction technology: techniques and results in a prospective study. Aesthet Surg J 2019. https://doi.org/10.1093/asj/sjz218.

6. The Art of BODY CONTOURING. The art of body contouring. 2017. https://doi.org/10.1055/b-0037-146533.

7. Fodor PB. Reflections on lipoplasty: history and personal experience. Aesthet Surg J 2009;29(3):226–31.

8. Illouz YG. Body contouring by lipolysis: a 5-year experience with over 3000 cases. Plast Reconstr Surg 1983;72(5):591–7.

9. Fodor PB, Vogt PA. Power-assisted lipoplasty (PAL): a clinical pilot study comparing PAL to traditional lipoplasty (TL). Aesthetic Plast Surg 1999;23(6):379–85.

10. Peter Rubin J, Jewell ML, Richter D, et al. Body contouring and liposuction E-book: expert consult - online. Edinburgh: Elsevier Health Sciences; 2012.

11. Mentz HA, Gilliland MD, Patronella CK. Abdominal etching: differential liposuction to detail abdominal musculature. Aesthetic Plast Surg 1993;17(4):287–90.

12. Hoyos AE, Millard JA. VASER-assisted high-definition liposculpture. Aesthet Surg J 2007;27(6):594–604.

13. Shiffman MA, Di Giuseppe A. Body contouring: art, science, and clinical practice. Berlin: Springer Science & Business Media; 2010.

14. Hoyos AE, Prendergast PM. High definition body sculpting. 2014. https://doi.org/10.1007/978-3-642-54891-8.

15. Frank K, Hamade H, Casabona G, et al. Influences of age, gender, and body mass index on the thickness of the abdominal fatty layers and its relevance for abdominal liposuction and abdominoplasty. Aesthet Surg J 2019. https://doi.org/10.1093/asj/sjz131.

16. Parashar S. Abdominal fat pathophysiology. Art of abdominal contouring: advanced liposuction. 2017:21-21. https://doi.org/10.5005/jp/books/12921_5.

17. Aly A, Nahas F. The art of body contouring: a comprehensive approach. New York: Thieme; 2017.

18. Bertheuil N, Chaput B, Berger-Müller S, et al. Liposuction preserves the morphological integrity of the microvascular network: flow cytometry and confocal microscopy evidence in a controlled study. Aesthet Surg J 2016;36(5):609–18.

19. Mendez BM, Coleman JE, Kenkel JM. Optimizing patient outcomes and safety with liposuction. Aesthet Surg J 2019;39(1):66–82.

20. Morris RJ, Woodcock JP. Evidence-based compression. Ann Surg 2004;239(2):162–71.

21. Husain TM, Salgado CJ, Mundra LS, et al. Abdominal etching: surgical technique and outcomes. Plast Reconstr Surg 2019;143(4):1051–60.

22. Wall SH Jr, Lee MR. Separation, aspiration, and fat equalization: SAFE liposuction concepts for comprehensive body contouring. Plast Reconstr Surg 2016;138(6):1192–201.

23. P. N. Ultrasound assisted liposculpture – UAL: a simplified safe body sculpturing and aesthetic beautification technique. Advanced Techniques in Liposuction and Fat Transfer. 2011. https://doi.org/10.5772/25146.

Deep Venous Thrombosis Prophylaxis

Casey T. Kraft, MD, Jeffrey E. Janis, MD*

KEYWORDS

- Abdominoplasty • Venous thromboembolism • VTE • DVT • PE • Deep venous thrombosis
- Pulmonary embolism • Prophylaxis

KEY POINTS

- Abdominoplasty has one of the highest risks for venous thromboembolism events in aesthetic surgery.
- Risk for venous thromboembolism is increased when concurrent intra-abdominal, circumferential, or liposuction procedures are performed with abdominoplasty. However, the data on abdominoplasty combined with liposuction are conflicting.
- There are no specific recommendations for venous thromboembolism risk reduction in abdominoplasty patients. Mechanical and chemical prophylaxis are at the discretion of the surgeon for each individual patient.
- The 2005 Caprini Thrombosis Risk Factor Assessment Form can be useful for risk stratification.

INTRODUCTION

Abdominoplasty is one of the most commonly performed aesthetic procedures in plastic surgery, with more than 130,000 procedures being performed in 2018.[1] Despite being one of the most popular plastic surgery procedures, there is a well-known increased risk of venous thromboembolism (VTE) consisting of deep venous thrombosis (DVT), pulmonary embolism (PE), or both, compared with other commonly performed aesthetic surgery procedures.[2]

Although the increased risk of abdominoplasty is well known, management of this risk is a contentious subject. The American Society of Plastic Surgeons (ASPS) has released general VTE prevention guidelines for plastic surgery procedures, but specific recommendations for higher-risk procedures such as abdominoplasty do not exist.[3] This omission leaves management up to individual surgeons, allowing a wide variation in practices for risk reduction.[4]

INCIDENCE

It is generally accepted that abdominoplasty has an increased risk of VTE events compared with other plastic surgery procedures. The exact risk varies by report in the literature because most articles published on the topic are retrospective reviews of large databases or cumulative data. A recent review of the literature with a combined statistical analysis reported the VTE rate for abdominoplasty alone at 0.34%, or 1 in 3000 procedures.[2] Another, more recent, study looked at VTE risk using the American Association for Accreditation of Ambulatory Surgery Facilities' Internet Based Quality Assurance Program database and reported an incidence of 0.06% for abdominoplasty alone.[5]

Abdominoplasty is frequently performed concurrently with other procedures, and this has been shown to confer additional risk for VTE. The amount of increased risk depends on the type of procedure performed, with additional risk primarily

Department of Plastic Surgery, The Ohio State University Wexner Medical Center, 915 Olentangy River Road, Suite 2100, Columbus, OH 43212, USA
* Corresponding author.
E-mail address: Jeffrey.Janis@osumc.edu

Clin Plastic Surg 47 (2020) 409–414
https://doi.org/10.1016/j.cps.2020.03.002
0094-1298/20/© 2020 Elsevier Inc. All rights reserved.

being conferred with intra-abdominal or circumferential procedures.[2,6,7] Abdominoplasty plus another concurrent plastic surgery procedure (not circumferential or intra-abdominal) does not seem to increase the risk of a VTE event compared with abdominoplasty alone.[2] In addition, this does not seem to depend on the number of concurrent procedures, with an additional 1 to 3 procedures reportedly having the same level of VTE risk.[5] The addition of liposuction to the abdominoplasty procedure may be an exception to this statement. The addition of liposuction specifically may increase the risk of a VTE event, although this topic has been greatly debated and reports are conflicting.[2,5,8]

More definitive evidence has shown that patients are subject to substantially higher risks of a VTE event when there is a concurrent intra-abdominal procedure performed with the abdominoplasty.[6] For patients undergoing abdominoplasty with a concurrent intra-abdominal procedure, the risk of a VTE event is estimated at 2.17%.[2] In addition, circumferential abdominoplasty (also known as belt lipectomy) confers a substantially increased risk of VTE events, estimated to be approximately 3.4%.[2] Surgeons and patients need to be knowledgeable of the risks of VTE events, particularly as they relate to concurrent procedures, in order to offer safe surgery and appropriate care postoperatively.

RISK STRATIFICATION
Potentially Modifiable Risk Factors

Given that abdominoplasty already presents a high risk for VTE events, surgeons must be aware of techniques and scoring models for patient risk stratification in order to inform proper decision making. Abdominoplasty is an elective surgery, providing surgeons with an opportunity to insist on modifiable risk factors being improved before operating. Nonmodifiable risk factors that are present may also need to be addressed preoperatively, which may best be accomplished by including other consultants in the patient workup before the operation in order to maximize patient safety.

The most commonly referenced and frequently studied score assessment model for VTE risk stratification is the 2005 Caprini Thrombosis Risk Assessment Model (**Fig. 1**).[9,10] The Caprini score is a weighted risk-assessment model that allows validated risk stratification based on numerous factors increasing the risk of a postoperative VTE event.[9]

Obtaining a preoperative Caprini score can be valuable for plastic surgeons to properly manage VTE risk postoperatively. Many of the risk factors included within the scoring model are potentially modifiable, and, for patients deemed high risk, insisting on lifestyle modification or other factors can dramatically change the individual's score. Some of the most notable modifiable components of the Caprini score are increased body mass index (>25), timing of surgery, oral contraceptive use, and recent pregnancy.[9] Previous studies have shown that a reduction of 1 to 2 points in a patient's Caprini score can cause a 2-fold to 4-fold decrease in the risk of a VTE event. This finding clearly shows that these modifiable factors can have a significant impact.[11] Recent studies by Pannucci and colleagues[12] suggest that effective prophylaxis with enoxaparin may require altering dosage depending on body weight rather than mere standard dosing. This work is preliminary and ongoing. For the nonmodifiable factors, elements such as previous history of DVT/PE or known hypercoagulable disorders may prompt a hematology consultation before surgery to ensure proper patient risk management. This decision should be up to the surgeon's discretion and each individual patient.

Surgical Factors Increasing Risk

Despite the modifiable risk factors present in many patients, there remain inherent risks with the abdominoplasty procedure. Historically, much of this risk has been attributed to rectus plication creating an increase in intra-abdominal pressure, resulting in venous stasis, a critical component of the Virchow triad.[13–15] However, more recent studies have evaluated abdominal pressures before and after rectus plication in abdominoplasty and found that the statistically significant increase in abdominal pressure was of questionable clinical significance.[16,17]

Other factors relatively specific to abdominoplasty that have been shown to increase abdominal pressure include skin closure, bed flexion, and the use of an abdominal binder postoperatively.[17] In addition, limited ambulation postoperatively because of pain, waist flexion, or any other factors may increase the risk of VTE events and should be avoided.[7,8,18] From a global perspective, surgeons should take all of these factors into consideration when performing abdominoplasty and adjust accordingly to reduce patient VTE risk as much as possible.

PREVENTION
Mechanical Prophylaxis

Little has been specifically studied regarding the use of mechanical prophylaxis in abdominoplasty. However, the ASPS has published a consensus

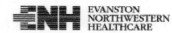

Thrombosis Risk Factor Assessment

Joseph A. Caprini, MD, MS, FACS, RVT
Louis W. Biegler Professor of Surgery,
Northwestern University
The Feinberg School of Medicine,
Professor of Biomedical Engineering,
Northwestern University;
Director of Surgical Research,
Evanston Northwestern Healthcare
Email: j-caprini@northwestern.edu
Website: venousdisease.com

Patient's Name:_____ Age: ____ Sex: ____ Wgt:____lbs

Choose All That Apply

Each Risk Factor Represents 1 Point

- ☐ Age 41–60 y
- ☐ Minor surgery planned
- ☐ History of prior major surgery (<1 mo)
- ☐ Varicose veins
- ☐ History of inflammatory bowel disease
- ☐ Swollen legs (current)
- ☐ Obesity (BMI >25)
- ☐ Acute myocardial infarction
- ☐ Congestive heart failure (<1 mo)
- ☐ Sepsis (<1 mo)
- ☐ Serious lung disease incl. pneumonia (<1 mo)
- ☐ Abnormal pulmonary function (COPD)
- ☐ Medical patient currently at bed rest
- ☐ Other risk factors_____

Each Risk Factor Represents 3 Points

- ☐ Age over 75 y
- ☐ History of DVT/PE
- ☐ **Family history of thrombosis[a]**
- ☐ Positive Factor V Leiden
- ☐ Positive Prothrombin 20210A
- ☐ Elevated serum homocysteine
- ☐ Positive lupus anticoagulant
- ☐ Elevated anticardiolipin antibodies
- ☐ Heparin-induced thrombocytopenia (HIT)
- ☐ Other congenital or acquired thrombophilia
  If yes:

Type_____
[a]most frequently missed risk factor

Each Risk Factor Represents 2 Points

- ☐ Age 60–74 y
- ☐ Arthroscopic surgery
- ☐ Malignancy (present or previous)
- ☐ Major surgery (>45 min)
- ☐ Laparoscopic surgery (>45 min)
- ☐ Patient confined to bed (>72 h)
- ☐ Immobilizing plaster cast (<1 mo)
- ☐ Central venous access

Each Risk Factor Represents 5 Points

- ☐ Elective major lower extremity arthroplasty
- ☐ Hip, pelvis or leg fracture (<1 mo)
- ☐ Stroke (<1 mo)
- ☐ Multiple trauma (<1 mo)
- ☐ Acute spinal cord injury (paralysis)(<1 mo)

For Women Only (Each Represents 1 Point)

- ☐ Oral contraceptives or hormone replacement therapy
- ☐ Pregnancy or postpartum (<1 mo)
- ☐ History of unexplained stillborn infant, recurrent spontaneous abortion (≥3), premature birth with toxemia or growth-restricted infant

Total Risk Factor Score ☐

Fig. 1. The 2005 Caprini Risk Assessment Model. [a]Most frequently missed risk factor. (*From* Caprini JA. Thrombosis risk assessment as a guide to quality patient care. Dis Mon. 2005; 51(2-3):70-78; with permission.)

statement recommending intermittent pneumatic compression stockings perioperatively for plastic surgery patients to reduce VTE risk.[19] They also specify that intermittent pneumatic compression stockings are superior to elastic compression stockings in the perioperative setting.[19] They do not provide recommendations for whether or not an extended duration of pneumatic compression stockings or elastic compression stockings is beneficial given a lack of publications on this topic. In a survey of 1106 plastic surgeons, Spring and colleagues[4] reported that most surgeons used intermittent pneumatic compression stockings for patients of all risk profiles (63% for low risk, 82% for moderate risk, and 85% for high risk). Although it may go beyond guideline recommendations, pneumatic compression stockings clearly are a commonly used method for VTE risk reduction in aesthetic surgery regardless of the patient's risk factors.[4,20]

Chemoprophylaxis

The use of chemoprophylaxis in abdominoplasty has been studied using a variety of different agents, including unfractionated heparin, low-

Table 1
Summary of the American Society of Plastic Surgeons venous thromboembolism task force recommendations

Step 1: Risk Stratification	
Patient Population	Recommendation
Inpatient: adult aesthetic and reconstructive plastic surgery patients who undergo general anesthesia	Should complete a 2005 Caprini Risk Factor Assessment Tool to stratify patients into a VTE risk category based on their individual risk factors. Grade B Or Should complete a VTE risk-assessment tool comparable with the 2005 Caprini RAM to stratify patients into a VTE risk category based on their individual risk factors. Grade D
Outpatient: adult aesthetic and reconstructive plastic surgery patients who undergo general anesthesia	Should consider completing a 2005 Caprini Risk Factor Assessment Tool to stratify patients into a VTE risk category based on their individual risk factors. Grade B Or Should consider completing a VTE risk-assessment tool comparable with the 2005 Caprini RAM to stratify patients into a VTE risk category based on their individual risk factors. Grade D

Step 2: Prevention		
Patient Population	2005 Caprini RAM Score	Recommendations[a]
Elective surgery patients (when the procedure is scheduled in advance and is not performed to treat an emergency or urgent condition)	≥7	Should consider using risk-reduction strategies such as limiting operating room times, weight reduction, discontinuing hormone replacement therapy, and early postoperative mobilization. Grade C
Patients undergoing the following major procedures when the procedure is performed under general anesthesia lasting more than 60 min: • Body contouring • Abdominoplasty • Breast reconstruction • Lower extremity procedures • Head/neck cancer procedures	3–6	Should consider the option to use postoperative LMWH or UH. Grade B

Abbreviations: LMWH, low-molecular-weight heparin; RAM, risk-assessment module; UH, unfractionated heparin.

[a] The scores associated with the recommendations apply to the 2005 Caprini risk-assessment module and were not intended for use with alternative VTE risk-assessment tools.

From Murphy R, Alderman A, Gutowski K, et al. Evidence-based practices for thromboembolism prevention: summary of the ASPS venous thromboembolism task force report. Plast Reconstr Surg. 2012; 130(1):168e-175e; with permission.

molecular-weight heparin, and oral anticoagulants such as rivaroxaban.[6,21–23] In general, the research is widely varied and with small sample sizes. In addition, most surgeons do not use chemoprophylaxis routinely, although the rate of usage is higher with high-risk patients.[4,5] However, previous studies have shown that there is a significant risk reduction with the use of chemoprophylaxis in high-risk plastic surgery patients without an increased risk of bleeding.[24] In addition, recent guidelines published in *JAMA* recommend low-molecular-weight heparin rather than unfractionated heparin, primarily in critically ill patients, although this may be less specific for plastic surgery outpatient procedures.[25] For abdominoplasty patients, other studies have shown that unfractionated heparin and low-molecular-weight heparin do not increase bleeding risk with perioperative administration, and they reduce the risk of VTE events in high-risk patients.[6,23]

For oral anticoagulants, most of the research has evaluated factor Xa inhibitors. These results are mixed. One small study reported a higher incidence of hematoma when using rivaroxaban, although dosages were not reported by the investigators.[26] Other studies have compared rivaroxaban and apixaban with lower-molecular-weight heparin for body contouring procedures and found similar rates of VTE events, along with similar (rivaroxaban and low-molecular-weight heparin) or lower (apixaban) rates of hematoma.[21] The largest study to date was a multicenter retrospective review of rivaroxaban prophylaxis for abdominoplasty with low rates of VTE events (0.76%) and hematomas (2.3%). Future studies are warranted to more fully evaluate the safety of oral anticoagulants for VTE prophylaxis, although initial results point toward its safety and efficacy.

FORMAL RECOMMENDATIONS

For situations such as abdominoplasty, a common aesthetic procedure with a higher risk of VTE events, surgeons often look to the literature for more formal recommendations to help decide on the most effective prophylaxis protocol, including form of prophylaxis and duration. However, no such guideline exists specifically for abdominoplasty. Surgeons must decide each patient's individual risk for thromboembolic events and create or adjust their protocols accordingly.

ASPS has released guidelines for VTE prophylaxis in plastic surgery patients, which can be a useful starting point for surgeons deciding on a postoperative protocol.[27] In a 2011 systematic literature review, the ASPS VTE task force focused specifically on the 2005 Caprini Risk Assessment Model rather than the 2010 model to avoid potentially overscoring patients for plastic surgery procedures.[3] After review, the task force found that there was not enough evidence to provide recommendations on specific prophylaxis medications, dosages, or durations, but it did provide a generalized guideline for when to risk stratify patients and when to consider additional prophylaxis (**Table 1**).

Note that, within the generalized guidelines for risk stratification, the task force specifically highlighted additional recommendations body contouring, abdominoplasty, breast reconstruction, lower extremity procedures, and head/neck cancer procedures.[27] These procedures were thought to be similar in risk to general surgery and orthopedic procedures given their anatomic location, degree of invasiveness, and similar patient population.[27] These specific situations have more detailed recommendations for prophylaxis considerations based on Caprini score than other plastic surgery procedures, and this should be taken into consideration for each abdominoplasty patient. One final caveat to these guidelines is that they were published in 2011, and novel oral anticoagulants such as dabigatran, rivaroxaban, and apixaban had only recently been US Food and Drug Administration approved and were not in common use at the time. Therefore, the use of these medications instead of enoxaparin or heparin for chemoprophylaxis is at the discretion of surgeons and their comfort with these medications and their risk profiles.

SUMMARY

Abdominoplasty is a commonly performed aesthetic procedure with a higher rate of VTE events compared with other aesthetic procedures. No abdominoplasty-specific guidelines exist for VTE prophylaxis, so surgeons should use previously published ASPS recommendations to risk stratify patients and treat them prophylactically based on their individual risk. Concurrent surgeries, particularly intra-abdominal procedures, seem to further increase risk. Mechanical prophylaxis is generally performed perioperatively, and all forms of chemoprophylaxis seem to be equivalent at this time, although more research is needed for newer-generation oral anticoagulants.

DISCLOSURE

Dr J.E. Janis has served as a prior consultant for LifeCell, Bard, Pacira, and Allergan within the last 12 months but has no current active affiliations. He receives royalties from Thieme Publishing. The remaining authors have no conflicts of interest to disclose. No funding was received for this research.

REFERENCES

1. Plastic surgery 2018 statistics report. Available at: https://www.plasticsurgery.org/documents/News/Statistics/2018/plastic-surgery-statistics-report-2018.pdf. Accessed September 1, 2019.
2. Hatef DA, Trussler AP, Kenkel JM. Procedural risk for venous thromboembolism in abdominal contouring surgery: a systematic review of the literature. Plast Reconstr Surg 2010;125(1):352–62.
3. Murphy RX Jr, Schmitz D, Rosolowski K. Evidence-based practices for thromboembolism prevention: a report from the ASPS venous thromboembolism

task force approved by ASPS executive committee. Plast Reconstr Surg 2012;130(1):168e–75e.

4. Spring MA, Gutowski KA. Venous thromboembolism in plastic surgery patients: survey results of plastic surgeons. Aesthet Surg J 2006;26(5):522–9.

5. Keyes GR, Singer R, Iverson RE, et al. Incidence and predictors of venous thromboembolism in abdominoplasty. Aesthet Surg J 2018;38(2):162–73.

6. Hatef DA, Kenkel JM, Nguyen MQ, et al. Thromboembolic risk assessment and the efficacy of enoxaparin prophylaxis in excisional body contouring surgery. Plast Reconstr Surg 2008;122(1):269–79.

7. Hurvitz KA, Olaya WA, Nguyen A, et al. Evidence-based medicine: abdominoplasty. Plast Reconstr Surg 2014;133(5):1214–21.

8. Friedland JA, Maffi TR. MOC-PS(SM) CME article: abdominoplasty. Plast Reconstr Surg 2008;121(4 Suppl):1–11.

9. Caprini JA. Thrombosis risk assessment as a guide to quality patient care. Dis Mon 2005;51(2–3):70–8.

10. Pannucci CJ. Venous thromboembolism in aesthetic surgery: risk optimization in the preoperative, intraoperative, and postoperative settings. Aesthet Surg J 2019;39(2):209–19.

11. Pannucci CJ, Bailey SH, Dreszer G, et al. Validation of the Caprini risk assessment model in plastic and reconstructive surgery patients. J Am Coll Surg 2011;212(1):105–12.

12. Pannucci CJ, Fleming KI, Bertolaccini C, et al. Double-blind randomized clinical trial to examine the pharmacokinetic and clinical impacts of fixed dose versus weight-based enoxaparin prophylaxis: a methodologic description of the FIxed or variable enoxaparin (FIVE) trial. Plast Reconstr Surg Glob Open 2019;7(4):e2185.

13. Hunter GR, Crapo RO, Broadbent TR, et al. Pulmonary complications following abdominal lipectomy. Plast Reconstr Surg 1983;71(6):809–17.

14. Jansen DA, Kaye AD, Banister RE, et al. Changes in compliance predict pulmonary morbidity in patients undergoing abdominal plication. Plast Reconstr Surg 1999;103(7):2012–5.

15. Kumar DR, Hanlin E, Glurich I, et al. Virchow's contribution to the understanding of thrombosis and cellular biology. Clin Med Res 2010;8(3–4):168–72.

16. Al-Basti HB, El-Khatib HA, Taha A, et al. Intraabdominal pressure after full abdominoplasty in obese multiparous patients. Plast Reconstr Surg 2004;113(7):2145–50 [discussion: 2151–5].

17. Huang GJ, Bajaj AK, Gupta S, et al. Increased intra-abdominal pressure in abdominoplasty: delineation of risk factors. Plast Reconstr Surg 2007;119(4):1319–25.

18. Somogyi RB, Ahmad J, Shih JG, et al. Venous thromboembolism in abdominoplasty: a comprehensive approach to lower procedural risk. Aesthet Surg J 2012;32(3):322–9.

19. Pannucci CJ, MacDonald JK, Ariyan S, et al. Benefits and risks of prophylaxis for deep venous thrombosis and pulmonary embolus in plastic surgery: a systematic review and meta-analysis of controlled trials and consensus conference. Plast Reconstr Surg 2016;137(2):709–30.

20. Harrison B, Khansa I, Janis J. Evidence-based strategies to reduce postoperative complications in plastic surgery. Plast Reconstr Surg 2016;137(1):351–60.

21. Morales R, Ruff E, Patronella C, et al. Safety and efficacy of novel oral anticoagulants vs low molecular weight heparin for thromboprophylaxis in large-volume liposuction and body contouring procedures. Aesthet Surg J 2016;36(4):440–9.

22. Hunstad JP, Krochmal DJ, Flugstad NA, et al. Rivaroxaban for venous thromboembolism prophylaxis in abdominoplasty: a multicenter experience. Aesthet Surg J 2016;36(1):60–6.

23. Campbell W, Pierson J, Cohen-Shohet R, et al. Maximizing chemoprophylaxis against venous thromboembolism in abdominoplasty patients with the use of preoperative heparin administration. Ann Plast Surg 2014;72(6):S94.

24. Seruya M, Venturi ML, Iorio ML, et al. Efficacy and safety of venous thromboembolism prophylaxis in highest risk plastic surgery patients. Plast Reconstr Surg 2008;122(6):1701.

25. Paul JD, Cifu AS. Prevention and management of venous thromboembolism. JAMA 2019. https://doi.org/10.1001/jama.2019.13853.

26. Dini GM, Ferreira MCC, Albuquerque LG, et al. How safe is thromboprophylaxis in abdominoplasty? Plast Reconstr Surg 2012;130(6):851e–7e.

27. Murphy RXJ, Alderman A, Gutowski K, et al. Evidence-based practices for thromboembolism prevention: summary of the ASPS venous thromboembolism task force report. Plast Reconstr Surg 2012;130(1):168e.

High-Definition Excisional Body Contouring
Mini Lipoabdominoplasty (FIT Mommy) and Enhanced Viability Abdominoplasty

Alfredo E. Hoyos Ariza, MD*, Mauricio E. Perez Pachon, MD

KEYWORDS

- Liposculpture • Abdominoplasty • Excisional surgery • Tummy tuck • Fat grafting • Liposuction
- High definition • Lipoplasty

KEY POINTS

- Scarring, pigmentation, and asymmetries remain important patient concerns when excisional abdominal surgery is performed and have become challenging for plastic surgeons.
- Full and mini lipoabdominoplasties can be combined with high-definition liposculpture to improve results and also ameliorate most of these stigmata.
- Enhanced viability abdominoplasty is a reproducible and safe procedure with very low rate of complications.
- Neoumbilicoplasty is a new and very useful concept to avoid hyperpigmentation issues, allowing us to enhance the youthful appearance of the abdominal area.
- FIT Mommy procedure is an option for those patients who benefit of some excision in the abdominal wall but do not need an entire resection.

INTRODUCTION

Body contouring procedures continue to increase in number worldwide, in part due to lifestyle changes, weight loss surgery, and social media pressures.[1] According to the 2018 American Society of Plastic Surgeons report on procedural statistics, tummy tuck (abdominoplasty) remains the fifth most common cosmetic procedure in the United States, with 130,081 cases.[2]

Years ago, surgeons realized that removing excess skin and fat tissue facilitated hernia repair and improved both the surgical result and patient satisfaction, as described in early lipectomy reports.[3] However, the proper term "abdominal lipectomy" was coined by Kelly in 1899, as the procedure was focused on adipose and skin flap resection.[4] Since these early descriptions, the technique has been subject to multiple modifications and technical improvements enhancing the surgical results.[5,6]

Recent publications have focused on technical variations and means of reducing surgical morbidity.[7,8]

Mini abdominoplasty was introduced by Greminger[9] in 1987 and Wilkinson[10] in 1988. They reported a case series of women with skin laxity and fat excess in the lower mid-region of the abdomen on whom a "limited" abdominoplasty was performed with very reliable results, However, the procedure was not widely adopted and full abdominoplasty remained the overwhelmingly most common option. Today indications for dermolipectomy in postpartum women are defined by the presence of stretch marks and/or laxity of

Funding: The authors received no financial support for the research, authorship, or publication of this article.
Dhara Clinic, Carrera 15 #83-33, Suite 304, Bogota, Colombia
* Corresponding author.
E-mail address: alhoyos@gmail.com
Twitter: @AlfredoHoyosMD (A.E.H.A.); @Maoperezmd (M.E.P.P.)

Clin Plastic Surg 47 (2020) 415–428
https://doi.org/10.1016/j.cps.2020.03.008

the skin. In patients with mild skin excess, a mini-lipectomy may be considered more appropriate, given the reduced morbidity and clear advantage of umbilicus preservation.

On the other hand, liposuction and newer technologies used alone or in conjunction with abdominoplasty have improved our results. Our experience includes the broad use of third-generation ultrasound (VASER, © 2018 Solta Medical - Bausch Health Companies Inc., Laval, Quebec, Canada) to perform selective fat emulsification, making fat extraction much easier, preserving flap vascularization, and improving long-term aesthetic results.[11] A detailed understanding of the 3-dimensional anatomy combined with new surgical tools allows the surgeon to sculpt the abdomen and reproduce the natural "lights and shadows" of the abdominal area. This forms the basis of high-definition lipoplasty techniques.[12] Although different techniques have been described, the major principles remain the same. The current authors have published their experience with 736 consecutive patients who underwent high-definition lipoabdominoplasty[13] as well

as the indications and results of patients who underwent mini-tummy tuck.[14]

In the next sections we will describe our experience with abdominoplasty techniques in addition to 360-degree high-definition liposculpture, which has allowed us to go beyond the traditional procedures.

Anatomy

The first important step during preoperative evaluation for body contour surgery is the detailed acknowledgment of the variable aspects of the individual's anatomy. The ideal abdomen is made of a complex combination of convexities and concavities created by the underlying muscle mass and bone prominences. In the female, the curvaceous, athletic, and slim appearance in the abdominal area is preferred, as this resembles youth and attractiveness. There are 3 areas of concavities recognized:

1. The subcostal area, between the lateral border of the rectus abdominis and the lower costal margin.

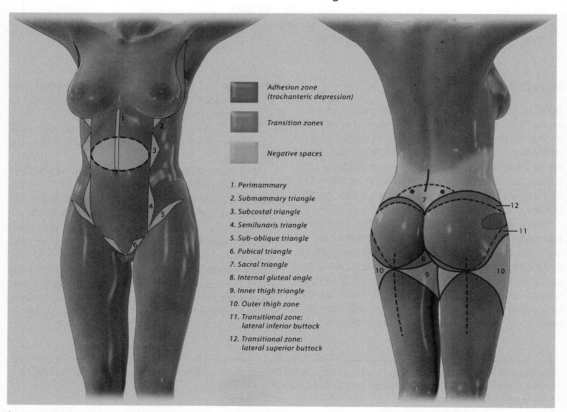

Adhesion zone
(trochanteric depression)

Transition zones

Negative spaces

1. Perimammary
2. Submammary triangle
3. Subcostal triangle
4. Semilunaris triangle
5. Sub-oblique triangle
6. Pubical triangle
7. Sacral triangle
8. Internal gluteal angle
9. Inner thigh triangle
10. Outer thigh zone
11. Transitional zone:
    lateral inferior buttock
12. Transitional zone:
    lateral superior buttock

Fig. 1. Negative spaces and transition zones for special framing. Triangles are marked for smooth definition in EVA and FIT Mommy procedures because they will restore the normal underlying anatomy with enhanced athletic and slim appearance.

2. Between the inguinal ligament and the lower border of the semilunaris line.
3. The midline above the umbilicus.

These concavities as well as other areas in the torso and lower back are special landmarks that we need to have in mind when performing body contour surgery in the abdominal area, as they will ensure the optimum and natural athletic look (**Fig. 1**).

Women experience different changes in their skin and abdominal wall during pregnancy, due to different mechanical, hormonal, immunologic, metabolic, and vascular changes. This includes pigment alterations, stretch marks, glandular hyper-function, acne and dermatitis, excessive connective tissue relaxation, and diastatic rectus abdominis muscles. Weight gain, skin laxity, and excess of selective fat deposits remain the principal characteristics in women postdelivery. On the other hand, women with excessive weight gain or some grade of obesity also experience some of these concerns. For these patients, to whom liposuction is not suitable because of the postoperative excess skin flap, evident stretch marks, and other issues described previously, excisional abdominal cosmetic surgery is indicated. A 360-degree high-definition liposculpture in addition to mini or full lipoabdominoplasties can be performed according to individual patient characteristics.

Variations among patients are multiple and complex, but the more the deformity the clearer and more aggressive the treatment should be. A detailed preoperative assessment will help to plan the appropriate procedure for each patient. Liposuction may be the best treatment for thin women with minor skin excess and fat deposits, whereas abdominoplasty is best for obese women with severe skin laxity, umbilical ptosis, and abundant abdominal fat deposits.

The difficult group to classify could be the patients who do not fit the criteria for liposuction or abdominoplasty, as they could be just "too little" and "too much," respectively. Today because of the emphasis on diet, health, and fitness, many women seeking abdominoplasty are less likely to be overweight. Also, more women are having their first pregnancy in their late 30s and early 40s under optimal conditions of medical care. As a consequence, these women require minimally invasive procedures with less obvious scars. So, we have considered these as specific indications for a minimum excisional procedure or FIT Mommy lipoabdominoplasty. On the other hand, there are some women who are marginal candidates for these procedures, but simply will not accept any other surgery (eg, due to large scars or risk concerns), making this technique a relative indication. These patients must be warned about the possibility of having suboptimal results.

The full abdominoplasty has constantly undergone new improvements reducing the complications associated with the procedure. Stigma about the umbilicus discoloration, and significant and obvious scarring make many think twice about undergoing such a procedure. In particular, the preoperative umbilicus position has been a controversial indication for mini versus full abdominoplasty. Different reports have attempted to standardize umbilical location but many differences exist among populations.[15] We have described an area rather than a unique position as follows[13]: First, we draw a point in the middle of the line between the xiphoid process and the pubic symphysis, then a second point in the intersection of the upper two-thirds and lower one-third of this same line. The zone limited by these 2 points is the one we consider would be optimal for umbilicus placement. In our experience, a straightforward indication for mini-tummy tuck should be the patient with a high umbilicus location and little supraumbilical skin redundancy. In

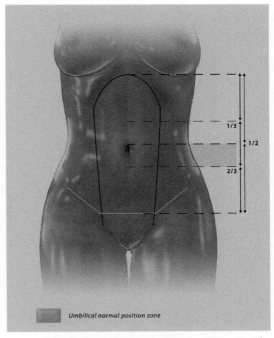

Fig. 2. Umbilical normal position zone. Area delimited over the midline (from the xiphoid process to the pubis) between the midpoint and the junction of the 2 upper thirds with a lower third. If the umbilicus is below this area, there is a high chance of requiring an EVA.

contrast, If the umbilicus was in or below the second drawn point, it would be a better candidate for a full lipoabdominoplasty.

Another important consideration regarding high-definition liposculpture is the *dynamic* concept of abdominal muscles. All of our muscles move and create different contours in our core structure, allowing our body to be in ceaseless motion. Abdominal muscles are constantly helping in the respiration process as well as the movement of the torso. This dynamic behavior has helped us design an aesthetic approach to avoid the standard "steady" appearance of the belly after liposuction, but rather improve the natural results in high-definition liposculpture. In abdominal excisional surgery, we always perform an active test of abdominal muscle contraction to determine the position of the rectus bellies and underlying anatomy of each patient. If we observe that the new umbilical position may be below the lower one-third of the xiphoid-pubic line, then a full abdominoplasty would be a better choice. Additional explanation is found in the markings section.

Neo Umbilicoplasty

The umbilicus shape and structure has been a matter of debate in multiple societies and cultures.

In fact, some religious beliefs surround this remnant of the umbilical cord. The umbilical scar is the foremost stigma that women worry about in lipoabdominoplasty. Its appearance changes through life due to aging and pregnancy: stretching, shape distortion (vertical to horizontal), presence of hernias, and hyperchromia due to hormonal changes in pregnancy may all occur.[16] These factors and its prime visible location give the umbilicus a very important role in abdominal aesthetics that should always be considered. Lipoabdominoplasty undoubtedly affects its position and shape on the abdominal wall. It almost always has a skin tone that is different from the surrounding skin after implantation. Performing a neoumbilicoplasty has consistently changed our patients' thoughts about full lipoabdominoplasty and has solved all these issues.

Gaudet and Morestin provided the first description of umbilical reconstruction in 1905; however, it was not until 1960 that the research focused on improving abdominal contour.[17] Pitanguy (1975),[18] Baroudi (1975),[19] Regnault (1975),[20] and Psillakis (1984)[21] highlighted the benefits of a lower location of the incision, making the umbilicus smaller and achieving acceptable long-term results. Hence, investigators have focused on describing different techniques for

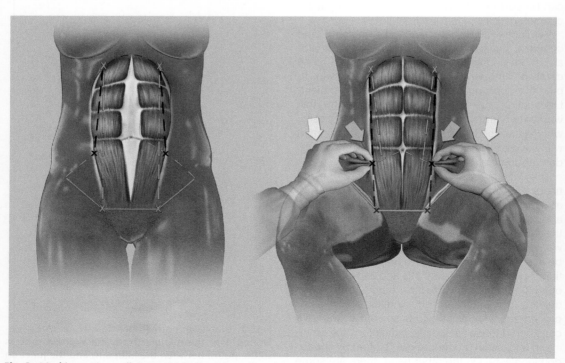

Fig. 3. Markings. Linea alba, actual (*left*) and predicted (*right*) positions are marked in resting position (*left*) and with active contraction (*right*). Active contraction helps us to predict the future position of the rectus abdominis muscle after plication.

neoumbilicoplasty and we have described our own, which we believe yields optimal results.[13,15]

With regard to umbilical placement, 3 main locations have been described in women: (1) a line drawn from xiphoid to pubis, the umbilicus is then located 60% of the distance from the xiphoid; (2) the umbilicus is located between the anterior-superior iliac spines[22]; (3) approximately 15 cm measured from the midpoint of the pubic bone upward.[23] These locations have been widely used among plastic and general surgeons in reconstructing and/or relocating the umbilicus. However, a standard measure has not yet been defined. We have considered the location as a dynamic concept that should fit the particularities of the patient's body distribution and height. So, the specific measures from pubis and iliac spines are not accurate because they do not take into account the height variations and/or the iliac shape. Because the xiphoid-pubis measurement varies according to the individual's height, youthfulness, and other anatomic considerations, we considered a better choice to describe an "umbilical zone" rather than a single point for each patient (**Fig. 2**).

SURGICAL TECHNIQUE
Enhanced Viability Abdominoplasty

According to the book of *Genesis* from the Bible, Eve was born form Adam's rib. However, as she did not have an umbilical cord, the umbilicus was nonexistent. This singular biblical deduction inspired us to create a full tummy-tuck procedure enhanced by VASER extraction that increases viability (enhanced viability abdominoplasty [EVA]) to perform high-definition liposculpture in addition to neoumbilicoplasty. It is conceived as a 3-phase procedure that starts with liposculpture, followed by abdominoplasty and ending with umbilicoplasty.

Markings
In standing position, general areas of extra fat deposits are marked on the trunk, abdomen, buttocks, thighs, and arms for deep liposuction. The negative zones for smooth liposuction are marked with another color following our own code. Prohibited zones are also marked in the gluteal and lumbar anatomic regions. The abdominal midline is marked by palpation of the linea alba. The surgeon must predict where the rectus abdominis muscle will be placed after plication. As we discussed previously, we must consider the dynamic concept of the muscular movement on the marking process: this should be done with the patient in a standing position paying attention to the

muscle insertions. Do not guide its markings by the superficial landmarks because of the muscular diastases caused by pregnancy. First, in resting muscular position we draw the muscle limits to determine the diastases zone; then, the patient is asked to perform an active muscle contraction to mark the upper and lower insertions of the rectus abdominis muscle. Once these points are referenced, a line is drawn from the upper to the lower direction to predict where the lateral border of the muscle is going to be placed after plication (**Fig. 3**).

Liposculpture Liposculpture is completed as a 3-step process:

1. Start in prone position and later in supine, with infiltration of tumescent solution (1000 mL of

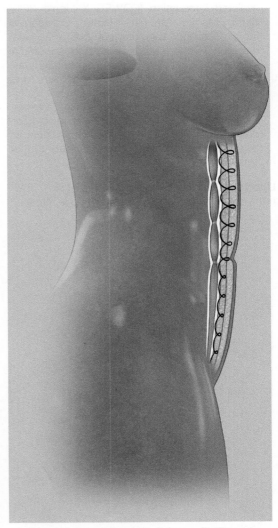

Fig. 4. Enhancing definition of the medial line: above the umbilicus very superficial stitching; below the umbilicus just grab the Scarpa fascia.

saline with additives of 10 mL of 1% lidocaine and 1 mL of epinephrine 1:1000) having a ratio of infiltration/removed volume of 2:1 to 1.5, approximately. We begin in the total prone position to perform a perfect symmetric and comparative liposculpture. By this time, the anesthesiologist makes ventilator changes to ensure a safe posterior liposuction always guided by CO_2 monitoring. Also, a fluid preoperative load of 10 to 15 cm^3/kg is administered to guarantee the cardiac preload and to minimize the hemodynamic effects of the prone position.

2. Fat emulsification is done by third-generation ultrasound (VASER) using 2-mm, 3-mm, and 3.7-mm grooved probes.

3. Extraction is performed using powered-assisted liposuction (POWER X Lipo© 2018 Solta Medical-Bausch Health Companies Inc.), following the preoperative markings, blending deep, intermediate, and superficial fat layers using 4.6-mm and 3.7-mm cannulas. The VASER is used in pulsed mode with 70 to 80 W for trunk and abdomen and 50 W for legs and arms. The harvested fat can be centrifuged and grafted in other zones (eg, gluteal, deltoid, and/or breast enhancement) as needed (see the *FIT Mommy* section for further explanation).

Lipectomy Beginning with a classic low-transverse incision, the abdominal flap is released in the lower abdomen in the sub-Scarpa layer and in the upper abdomen in the suprafascial level, using a tunneling technique with careful hemostatic control followed by plication of the rectus abdominis muscles. The native umbilicus is resected, and the remnant is fixed to the deep fascia. The abdominal flap is then advanced and secured with a progressive tension technique; wide continuous stitches are used from the xiphoid down to the umbilicus (progressive tension suture) to enhance the midline appearance in the upper abdomen using absorbable suture. Below the umbilicus, the stitching is made less superficial than above, just grabbing Scarpa fascia (**Fig. 4**). The excess skin is then resected, and closure is performed in layers. A single closed Jackson-Pratt drain is placed at the end of the procedure (Blake ETHICON, Inc., Johnson & Johnson, Cincinnati, OH). Any additional liposuction over the flap is then performed following the markings to enhance the muscular definition.

Neoumbilicoplasty: immediate versus delayed
Although not conventional, delayed neoumbilicoplasty may be necessary to preserve the flap viability. The choice is made intraoperatively according to the following conditions: (1) high flap tension; (2) flap discoloration or congestion; (3) thick flap, which required more liposuction over the area; (4) if additional definition was performed or planned for a second procedure; (5) inadequate flap descent or if inverted T-flap closure was

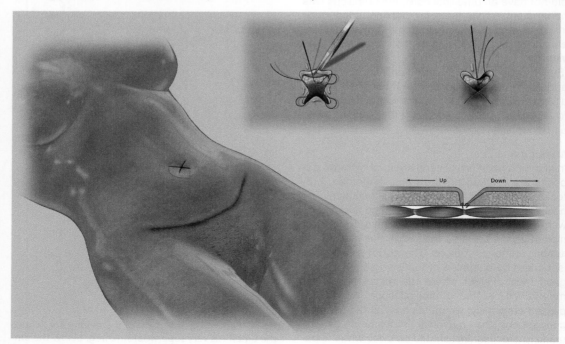

Fig. 5. Neoumbilicoplasty. Butterfly technique: X-shaped incision with upper larger flaps.

necessary; (6) secondary or revision lipectomy; (7) high scar placement. The timing for the neoumbilicoplasty procedure is defined by the time the drain is removed after the first stage (7–10 days). Some patients chose to do the navel procedure after feeling completely healed of the lipoabdominoplasty (4–8 weeks). The ideal umbilical zone is the area delimited over the midline (from the xyphoid process to the pubis) between the midpoint and the junction of the 2 upper thirds with a lower third (see **Fig. 2**). Within this line, the umbilicus should be placed according to the height of the patient in a higher or lower position. Higher locations are preferable in younger patients, fit women, and patients who want an

athletic look. The lower location is preferable in older patients, women who want a rather "soft" (nonathletic) look, or patients with larger and/or ptotic breasts (ptotic breasts tend to make the optical illusion of a shorter torso). After defining the best location for the umbilicus, zones for deep and superficial liposuction can be marked for extra fat resection and definition when delayed neoumbilicoplasty is performed.

Neoumbilicoplasty procedure
An X-shaped incision, with 60° in the apex angles, is done across the linea alba, deep enough to reach the rectus abdominis fascia. Upper incisions must be 10 mm long and lower incisions 5 mm. As

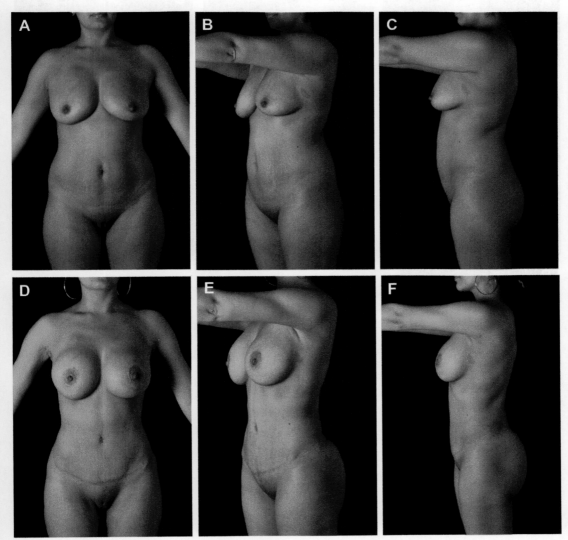

Fig. 6. A 36-year-old woman. EVA was performed. Observe the new athletic and youthful appearance of the abdomen in addition to a low scar placement in the postoperative pictures (*D–F*) compared with the preoperative pictures (*A–C*).

a result, 4 triangular flaps appear: superior, inferior, left, and right. The 3 lower flaps are sutured with continuous subcuticular stitch and fixed upward to the abdominal fascia in a spot located on the base of the upper flap (**Fig. 5**). The superior flap is fixed loosely to the fascia, in a perpendicular way. The wound is covered with gauze embedded in topical antibiotic to induce a round umbilicus shape. After week 1, the gauze is removed and a silicone spherical splint or a marble is left in the umbilical hole for 2 more weeks.

Postoperative Patients with fat extraction of more than 5000 mL, tense or high-risk flap, additional procedures, and comorbidities, such as hypertension or diabetes, are eligible for overnight in-hospital observation. A loose garment and a foam vest are indicated to use from the immediate postoperative period until 8 weeks. Patients are recommended to sleep in supine or lateral position as tolerated. Prone position is not recommended to protect the flap and avoid the neoumbilicus flattening. Follow-up visits are done at 48 hours postoperative and 3, 6, and 12 months. Photo records are made in each of the preoperative and postoperative appointments (**Figs. 6** and **7**). Postoperative CARE program is recommended for all our patients. This program includes lymphatic

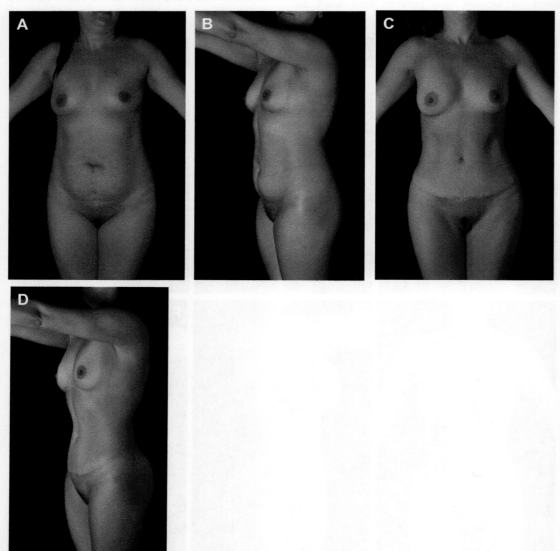

Fig. 7. A 40-year-old female patient. EVA was performed. Notice the preoperative (*A, B*) low position of the umbilicus and the abundant pannus surrounding the abdominal area. After EVA (*C, D*), the new slim figure and higher-positioned umbilicus makes the patient look younger.

drainage, massage therapy, active and passive physical therapy, and ultrasound. Trained nurses and therapists are carefully instructed in structured protocols.

Complications Although strict protocols and safely procedures are planned in each of our patients, every surgeon is likely to face some complications related to these procedures. Most are associated with uncontrollable variables, whereas others may be associated with technical errors.

Minor complications, such as seroma, prolonged bruising, and swelling, are the most common complications (6%–7%), usually occurring after drain removal. All of them can be solved with local therapy and external ultrasonic therapy (3 MHz). Less frequent complications include infections, bleeding, flap necrosis, and/or fat necrosis (2%–3%). In almost all cases, flap loss should be treated conservatively with debridement, local wound care, and healing by secondary intention. In our series,[13] delayed umbilicoplasty was associated with a decreased incidence of flap problems.

Mini Lipoabdominoplasty (FIT Mommy)

Some patients are not suitable for a full lipoabdominoplasty because of limited skin excess, but liposculpture appears to be insufficient. This is why we described the dynamic definition mini lipoabdominoplasty.[14] The procedure was designed for those patients who needed a little abdominal fat pad resection as well as high-definition liposculpture to achieve optimal results.

Markings

Markings for fat removal and abdominoplasty are identical to what was described for EVA. To predict where the rectus abdominis muscles are going to be located after the surgical procedure, the superior and inferior insertions of the rectus abdominis are marked in contraction, and a continuous line is drawn between these 2 points. These lines are called dynamic lines, as they recreate the active movement of the muscle (**Fig. 8**).

High-definition liposculpture Once the patient is marked, we start liposculpture by performing

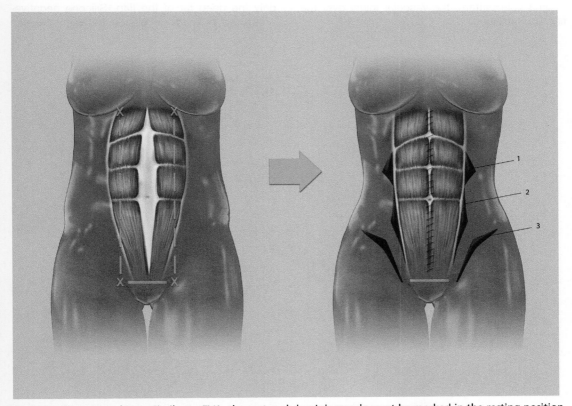

Fig. 8. FIT Mommy makings. Similar to EVA, the rectus abdominis muscle must be marked in the resting position (*left*) and in active contraction (*right*) to predict the position of the lateral border after plication. Additional definition of the subcostal (1), semilunaris (2) and suboblique (3) triangles could be done if necessary. Remember that general markings (negative spaces and transition zones) must be made for a 360-degree procedure.

stealth incisions (4–5 mm) over hidden anatomic creases and grooves (eg, posterior axillary fold, elbow crease, infragluteal and intergluteal crease, inframammary fold, and the supra pubic region medial to the lateral border of the rectus abdominis muscle). Silicone ports are fixed over the incisions and each area is infiltrated with standard tumescent solution (1000 mL of normal saline, 20 mL 1% lidocaine, and 1 ampoule of epinephrine 1:1000), in the superficial and deep fat layers. Fat emulsification is performed with third-generation ultrasound (VASER), blended between the superficial, intermediate, and deep fat layers with 3.7-mm 2-ring probes. In the superficial and intermediate layer, VASER is used in 80% pulsed mode, whereas in the deep layer it is used in 80% continuous mode. Deep lipoplasty is performed in the lateral and mid region of the abdomen using 3.0-mm and 3.7-mm long cannulas. The waistline area is suctioned by 4.6-mm, 3.0-mm curved, and semi-curved cannulas. Superficial lipoplasty is performed for definition of the rectus (the predicted lines, or dynamic lines) and oblique abdominal muscles with the alba line, with small cannulas (3.0, 3.7 mm). By using a small-diameter, low-trauma hole pattern, the vascular injury over the flap is diminished.

Mini lipoabdominoplasty After liposuction, a transverse incision over the supra pubic region is made, in the same position as the Pfannenstiel technique described for cesarean surgery.[24] The fold over the pubis marks the horizontal section of the skin in the superior border of the pubic hair, following a convex curved line, 10 to 12 cm long. The anterior abdominal flap is raised from the pubic incision to the xiphoid process, releasing the umbilicus from its base to access the upper abdominal flap. Hemostasis is carefully done in the flap and the rectus abdominis muscle is plicated in 2 layers: double x stitches and later a running suture (absorbable). The plication is carefully performed, avoiding overcorrection of the muscle, otherwise the definition will fall in a nonanatomic place and might look like a "double" rectus abdominis muscle. If more plication were needed, then transverse muscle plication could be performed bilaterally in the lower abdomen (**Fig. 9**).

Finally, the flap and the umbilicus are fixed to the muscular fascia with absorbable running suture. In the upper abdomen, the running suture must grab the dermis of the flap to increase the definition, whereas in the lower abdomen the stitches include only the deep fat of the flap. Silicone negative-pressured drainage is placed between the flap

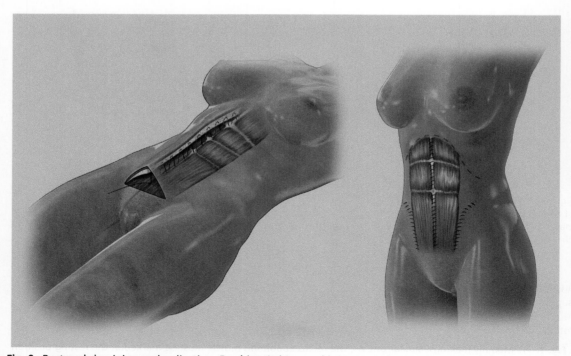

Fig. 9. Rectus abdominis muscle plication. Double stitching and later a running suture are performed to define the linea alba. Transverse muscle plication could be performed bilaterally for additional definition if requested by the patient.

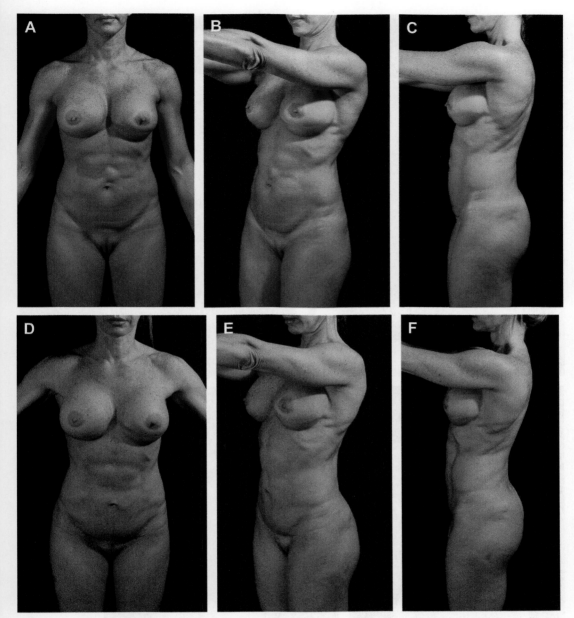

Fig. 10. A 44-year-old woman. This patient's athletic preoperative state (*A–C*) is affected by postdelivery diastases of the rectus abdominis muscle and an evident supraumbilical hernia. FIT Mommy procedure allowed us to primarily correct the wall defect and improve the athletic and muscular appearance of the abdomen after muscle plication (*D–F*).

and the fascia. The closure is made from deep to superficial layers, excess fat and skin tissue is removed, and the wound sutured. Deep layer aspiration could be done for further debulking. Superficial layer aspiration completes the procedure to define athletic depressions, such as the linea alba, the lateral borders of the rectus, and the oblique muscles.

Fat grafting

Fat harvesting was made with a 3-mm blunt cannula to an empty, sterile bottle trap with 1 g of cefazolin added. Decantation process was achieved for fat-cell separation from the saline and serum and blood components. The high-density supernatant was fully recovered for selective fat grafting. Lipoinjection was performed with

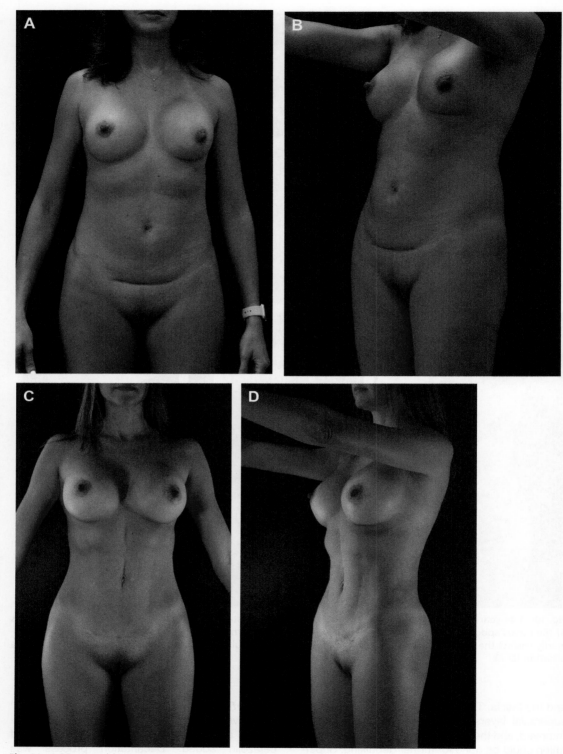

Fig. 11. A 38-year-old woman. FIT Mommy was performed. The postoperative scar is almost invisible and the new athletic and slim shape of the abdomen (*C, D*) has completely changed, compared with the preoperative appearance (*A, B*).

a 3-mm blunt cannula, to restore the aesthetically pleasant anatomy, distributed in hips, buttocks, deltoids, and calves. Zones lacking projection or desired for augmentation were grafted in the subcutaneous and/or intramuscular layers (**Figs. 10 and 11**).

Postoperative care Postoperative care is identical to the EVA procedure.

Complications Minor and major complications are similar although less frequent than those associated with the EVA technique. Skin burns are prone to occur if not correctly advised when performing VASER emulsification. Constant movement of the tip of the cannula and wet towels near ports help to prevent them. If present, each patient must be individualized and treated according to the type of lesion. Asymmetries might also occur if adequate markings are not performed or followed intraoperatively. Constant comparison in the operating room and an experienced surgeon makes such problems rare.

DISCUSSION

EVA lipoabdominoplasty was designed to address the pitfalls described by Lockwood[25] and expanded by the observation of traditional techniques. The use of internal ultrasonic devices combined with low-trauma–designed cannulas allows us to achieve: (1) better lateral abdominal superficial and deep liposuction, creating a defined waistline and lateral skin retraction; (2) deep liposuction and superficial ultrasonic release of the central flap, which addresses the tension over the central flap, migration, and hypertrophic scars and the pubic hair displacement; and (3) muscular definition creating the natural concavities of the abdomen, avoiding the "tense"-looking abdomen. How to deal with patients with large amounts of intra-abdominal fat remains an unanswered question. Extra fat resection over the upper abdomen would endanger the flap, as well as a tighter upper abdominal plication increases the risk plication failure and of increasing intra-abdominal pressure.

Large liposuction volume extraction (>5000 cm^3) with flap resection has been associated with blood loss resulting in anemia; however, transfusions are considered only when there are symptoms of anemia (ie, tachycardia, low blood pressure, headache, dizziness, and weakness).

The implementation of a neoumbilicoplasty technique mostly resolves major conventional abdominoplasty concerns. We can choose the umbilical position, short distance between the navel and the scar is not a problem. An inverted T lipectomy scar can be pulled down and converted in a linear scar while doing a delayed neoumbilicoplasty, leaving a better scar and navel position. Umbilical scarring either with larger than normal navel or constricted scar, navel hyperchromia, and residual umbilical hernias are rarely of concern; however, the neoumbilicoplasty may create a new kind of pitfall. Neo umbilical failure can occur. Fortunately, a new neoumbilicoplasty can be done later. Although umbilical reconstruction delay is not standard practice, it may be necessary in cases of questionable flap viability.

EVA is a safe and reproducible technique to perform abdominoplasty with the advantage of the high-definition liposculpture outcomes. Aesthetically pleasing results can be achieved and an athletic contour can be accomplished when desired.

Fit Mommy tuck is a new approach for those patients who do not meet criteria for EVA but do need some kind of excisional procedure. Some reports have described a partial abdominoplasty or "limited abdominoplasty," but for some women this might not be the best aesthetic solution. This new technique is easily learned, reproducible, and results in less morbidity. In selected patients it provides a better aesthetic outcome than a full abdominoplasty.

DISCLOSURE

The authors did not have financial interest nor receive any financial support of the products or devices mentioned in this article. All other authors declare that they have no conflicts of interest.

CONFLICTS OF INTEREST

Dr A.E. Hoyos was an unpaid consultant and speaker for the product development team of Sound Surgical Technologies (SST) system and cannulas (now: VASER© 2018 Solta Medical - Bausch Health Companies Inc.) up to May 2013. He receives royalties for the liposuction kits named after him.

REFERENCES

1. Watson A, Murnen SK, College K. Gender differences in responses to thin, athletic, and hypermuscular idealized bodies. Body Image 2019;30: 1–9.
2. Cosmetic Surgery National Data Bank STATISTICS. Available at: https://www.surgery.org/sites/default/files/ASAPS-Stats2018.pdf. Accessed September 10, 2019.
3. Regnault P. The history of abdominal dermolipectomy. Aesthet Plast Surg 1978;2(1):113–23.

4. Shiffman MA, Mirrafati S. Abdominoplasty History and Techniques (Ch 4). In: Aesthetic Surgery of the Abdominal Wall. Berlin: Springer; 2010.

5. Matarasso A. Abdominolipoplasty: a system of classification and treatment for combined abdominoplasty and suction-assisted lipectomy. Aesthet Plast Surg 1991;15:111.

6. Illouz YG. A new safe and aesthetic approach to suction abdominoplasty. Aesthet Plast Surg 1992; 16(3):237–45.

7. Boudreault DJ, Sieber DA. Getting the best results in abdominoplasty: current advanced concepts. Plast Reconstr Surg 2019;143(3):628e–36e.

8. Brauman D, van der Hulst RRWJ, van der Lei B. Liposuction assisted abdominoplasty: an enhanced abdominoplasty technique. Plast Reconstr Surg Glob Open 2018;6(9):e1940.

9. Greminger RF. The Mini-Abdominoplasty. Plastic and Reconstructive Surgery 1987;79(3):356–64.

10. Wilkinson TS. Mini-Abdominoplasty. Plastic and Reconstructive Surgery 1988;82(5):917.

11. Saldanha OR, Azevedo SF, Delboni PS, et al. Lipoabdominoplasty: the Saldanha technique. Clin Plast Surg 2010;37(3):469.

12. Hoyos AE, Prendergast PM. High definition body sculpting: art and advanced lipoplasty techniques. Berlin: Springer; 2014.

13. Hoyos A, Perez ME, Guarin DE, et al. A report of 736 high-definition lipoabdominoplasties performed in conjunction with circumferential VASER liposuction. Plast Reconstr Surg 2018;142(3):662–75.

14. Hoyos AE, Perez ME, Castillo L. Dynamic definition mini-lipoabdominoplasty combining multilayer liposculpture, fat grafting, and muscular plication. Aesthet Surg J 2013;33(4):545–60.

15. Joseph WJ, Sinno S, Brownstone ND, et al. Creating the perfect umbilicus: a systematic review of recent literature. Aesthet Plast Surg 2016;40(3):372–9.

16. Nussbaum R, Benedetto AV. Cosmetic aspects of pregnancy. Clin Dermatol 2006;24:133–41.

17. Pitanguy I. Surgical reduction of the abdomen, thigh, and buttocks. Surg Clin North Am 1971; 51(2):479–89.

18. Pitanguy I. Abdominal lipectomy. Clin Plast Surg 1975;2(3):401–10.

19. Baroudi R. Umbilicoplasty. Clin Plast Surg 1975;2(3): 431–48.

20. Regnault P. Abdominal dermolipectomies. Clin Plast Surg 1975;2(3):411–29.

21. Psillakis JM. Plastic surgery of the abdomen with improvement in the body contour. Physiopathology and treatment of the aponeurotic musculature. Clin Plast Surg 1984;11(3):465–77.

22. Suhas V, Anirudha G, Prajakta A. Anatomical localization of the umbilicus: an Indian Study. Plast Reconstr Surg 2006;117:1153.

23. Rodriguez-Feliz J, Makhijani S, Przybyla A, et al. Intraoperative assessment of the Umbilicopubic distance: a reliable anatomic landmark for transposition of the umbilicus. Aesthet Plast Surg 2012;36(1):8–17.

24. Decarle DW, Durfee RB. The Pfannenstiel incision for cesarean section. West J Surg Obstet Gynecol 1948;56(6):360–4.

25. Lockwood T. High-Lateral-Tension Abdominoplasty with Superficial Fascial System Suspension. Plastic and Reconstructive Surgery 1995;96(3):603–15.

Measuring Outcomes in Cosmetic Abdominoplasty
The BODY-Q

Claire E.E. de Vries, MD[a],*, Anne F. Klassen, DPhil[b],
Maarten M. Hoogbergen, MD, PhD[c], Amy K. Alderman, MD, MPH[d],
Andrea L. Pusic, MD, MSc[a]

KEYWORDS

- Abdominoplasty • Body contouring • Outcomes • Quality of life
- Patient-reported outcome measures • Aesthetic surgery

KEY POINTS

- Surgeons performing cosmetic abdominoplasty strive for high levels of patient satisfaction and improved quality of life for their patients.
- The BODY-Q is a comprehensive patient-reported outcome measure designed to measure outcomes relevant to cosmetic body contouring patients, as well as bariatric and massive weight loss patients, which can be used to measure the impact of cosmetic abdominoplasty procedures from the patient's perspective.
- Measuring surgical outcomes in an objective and reliable manner will help inform both patients and surgeons of the impact of different types of elective abdominal contouring procedures.

INTRODUCTION

Abdominoplasty is one of the most common cosmetic procedures performed worldwide. According to the American Society for Aesthetic Plastic Surgery, approximately 160,000 cosmetic abdominoplasty procedures were performed in the United States in 2018, a 170% increase since 2000.[1,2] Abdominoplasty is not just growing in volume but also in diversity of types of abdominoplasty procedures.[3,4] This procedure is performed in a diverse patient population (ranging from postpartum women to weight loss patients), which has led to a wide range of different surgical techniques, each with specific indications.[3–5] As more surgical techniques develop, a strong evidence-based guide in selecting the most appropriate procedure for each patient is necessary.[6,7] Surgeons need scientifically sound and clinically meaningful data to make informed medical decisions, and patients may benefit from these data by better understanding the expected outcomes and having a more active role in surgical decision making.

Cosmetic abdominoplasty procedure outcomes can be evaluated by using clinical end points such as complications and patient-reported outcomes (PROs) that measure health-related quality of life

Funding: The qualitative phase (phase I) of the BODY-Q study was funded by a research grant received from the Plastic Surgery Foundation (120593). The international field-test was funded by a grant from the Canadian Institutes for Health Research (CIHR). Dr A. Pusic received support through the NIH/NCI Cancer Center Support Grant P30 CA008748. In addition, A. Klassen held a CIHR Mid-Career Award in Women's Health.
[a] Department of Surgery, Brigham and Women's Hospital, 75 Francis Street, Boston, MA, USA; [b] McMaster University, 3N27, 1280 Main Street West, Hamilton, Ontario L8N 3Z5, Canada; [c] Department of Plastic and Reconstructive Surgery, Catharina Hospital, Michelangelolaan 2, Eindhoven 5623 EJ, the Netherlands; [d] North Atlanta Plastic Surgery, 3180 North Point Parkway, Suite 530, Alpharetta, GA 30005, USA
* Corresponding author.
E-mail addresses: cdevries@bwh.harvard.edu; devries.cee@gmail.com

(HR-QOL). Traditionally, there has been a strong emphasis on clinical outcomes.[8] However, because the main goal of abdominoplasty is to optimize appearance and HR-QOL, clinical data are insufficient on their own to evaluate the effectiveness of abdominoplasty procedures. Although clinical data remain important, they do not provide insight into patients' perspectives regarding the outcomes of surgery. PRO data take into account the patient's viewpoint, which adds an important perspective to the assessment of surgical procedures. PROs are best assessed by means of PRO measures (PROMs) and can be useful in clinical decision making and in comparative effectiveness research.[9]

PROMs are used not only in academic and industry-funded research but can also be used by individual cosmetic surgeons in clinical practice. Advancements in technology have made it feasible to collect PROMs data electronically, which can provide immediate display of results.[10] Surgeons can gain real-time insight into patients' self-reported outcomes. Collected in advance of an appointment, such information can then be used to prepare clinic visits by identifying health needs or concerns.[11] The use of PROMs can enhance the interactions between patients and surgeons, such as helping patients verbalize their feelings, and thereby supporting shared treatment decision making. Preoperatively, PROMs can help to screen patients who may have underlying psychological issues and require additional referral or support, or to identify patients who may require education to ensure realistic expectations about the outcomes that can be achieved. In previous studies, PRO data collection in clinical practice has been associated with increased frequency of patients discussing their outcomes, improved symptom control, and satisfaction with care.[12–14]

Despite the interest in using PROMs in cosmetic abdominoplasty, PRO data have not been rigorously and comprehensively collected. In the absence of PROMs specific to the abdominoplasty population, generic PROMs (ie, the Short Form 36) have been the most frequently used measures.[15–18] Generic PROMs are designed for general use not related to a specific disease or condition and can be used for comparison of HR-QOL across different patient populations or with healthy controls. However, generic PROMs lack domains relevant specifically to patients undergoing abdominoplasty procedures (eg, scarring related to body contouring procedures). Furthermore, generic PROMs may be limited by lack of sensitivity to measure changes (ie, responsiveness) as a result of not asking questions most relevant to cosmetic abdominoplasty patients.

PROMs specific to the abdominoplasty population are able to detect differences that occur after surgery, and these measures should be used to evaluate the effectiveness of surgical procedures.

Systematic Review

In order for PROMs to be meaningfully used in cosmetic abdominoplasty, it is essential to identify the most appropriate PROMs for this patient population. To appropriately measure the impact of abdominoplasty, PROMs should be valid, reliable, and sensitive with regard to detecting the effects of abdominoplasty on outcomes over time. Most importantly, a PROM should have content validity, which means that the content should be relevant, comprehensive, and comprehensible.[19] For example, if a PROM has 10 items, but 5 do not apply to the patient population, the scale will not be as effective in measuring outcomes. Similarly, if relevant issues were missed from the scale, or items are worded in a way that is not easy to understand and answer, these issues also reduce the effectiveness of the PROM. A well-developed PROM enables surgeons to understand the value of abdominoplasty procedures from the patients' perspective. In a systematic review to identify PROMs available in body contouring surgery, 2 different PROMs were found that had undergone development and validation in a body contouring surgery population.[20] Of these 2 PROMs, the BODY-Q was determined to be the most scientifically sound.[20] The BODY-Q was supported by evidence of sufficient measurement properties.[21–23] Most importantly, the BODY-Q showed excellent content validity, which describes that the items of the BODY-Q were relevant, comprehensive, and comprehensible.[19,24] The involvement of patients throughout the development of the BODY-Q ensured that outcomes most important to them were included in the BODY-Q.

THE BODY-Q

The BODY-Q is a comprehensive PROM designed to measure outcomes relevant to cosmetic body contouring patients, as well as bariatric and massive weight loss patients.[21,25,26] The BODY-Q conceptual framework consists of 3 domains (appearance, HR-QOL, and patient experience of health care) that can be measured using 25 independently functioning scales (Table 1).[21,24–26] Each scale represents a standalone instrument. The modular approach enables researchers or clinicians to select the BODY-Q scale that is most relevant to their research or clinical purposes.

Table 1
Overview of the domains and scales of the BODY-Q

Domain	Scale	Items	Example Item	Response Option Format
Appearance	Body	10	How your body looks when you are dressed	Dissatisfied/satisfied
	Abdomen	7	How your clothes fit your abdomen	Dissatisfied/satisfied
	Arms	7	The size of your upper arms	Dissatisfied/satisfied
	Back	4	How smooth your back looks	Dissatisfied/satisfied
	Buttocks	5	The size of your buttocks	Dissatisfied/satisfied
	Cellulite	11	How the skin where you have cellulite looks (not as smooth as you would like)	Not at all/extremely bothered
	Hips and outer thighs	5	The size of your hips and outer thighs	Dissatisfied/satisfied
	Inner thighs	4	How smooth your inner thighs look	Dissatisfied/satisfied
	Chest	10	How your chest (breast area) looks in a loose T-shirt	Dissatisfied/satisfied
	Nipples	5	The shape of your nipples?	Dissatisfied/satisfied
	Stretchmarks	10	Not being able to wear certain clothes because of your stretch marks	Not at all/extremely bothered
	Skin	7	Your excess skin making you look bigger than you are (ie, overweight)	Not at all/extremely bothered
	Scars	10	Having to dress in a way to hide your scars	Not at all/extremely bothered
Health-related Quality of Life	Body image	7	I feel positive toward my body	Agree/disagree
	Physical	7	Getting up from a bed	All the time/never
	Psychological	10	I believe in myself	Agree/disagree
	Sexual	5	Sex is fulfilling for me	Agree/disagree
	Social	10	I feel at ease at social gatherings with people I know	Agree/disagree
	Appearance-related psychosocial distress	8	I feel unhappy about how I look	Agree/disagree
Experience of health care	Doctor	10	Acted in a professional manner	Agree/disagree
	Office staff	10	Treated you with respect	Agree/disagree
	Medical team	10	Made sure to protect your privacy	Agree/disagree
	Information	10	The amount of written information they gave you to read	Dissatisfied/satisfied
	Expectations	8	I will look fantastic	Agree/disagree

The BODY-Q scales were developed in a 3-phase mixed-methods approach following rigorous guidelines for instrument development (ie, reports from the Scientific Advisory Committee of the Medical Outcomes Trust, the US Food and Drug Administration [FDA], and Consensus-based Standards for the Selection of Health Measurement Instruments [COSMIN] checklist).[27–30] The 3 phases were item generation, item reduction, and psychometric evaluation, and these phases have been published elsewhere.[21,24–26] In the first phase, the conceptual framework, preliminary scales, and items were generated from a literature review and were further augmented with 63 in-depth patient interviews.[24] Patient quotations from the patient interviews were used to generate preliminary items for the BODY-Q. Patients and professionals were asked about the relevance, comprehensiveness, and/or comprehensibility of the items of the BODY-Q. Feedback from 3 rounds of cognitive interviews with 22 participants and expert input were used to revise the scales to ensure that all relevant items were included in each construct of the different BODY-Q scales. Each BODY-Q item includes 4 response options, and patients provided feedback on the appropriateness of these response options. In the second phase, an international and multicenter field-test study was performed with 734 patients recruited. The data were analyzed to reduce the number of items in each scale.[21] The BODY-Q was analyzed using Rasch measurement theory (RMT), a modern psychometric approach. By using RMT analysis, items were selected that could be grouped together to form a valid BODY-Q scale. The questions in the BODY-Q scales were arranged in a meaningful, hierarchical order. As an example, the first item in the physical function scale is "Getting up from a bed," which is considered an easy measure of physical function to endorse. Further along the scale, the last question in the scale asks about "Standing for a long period of time," which is considered a difficult question of physical function to endorse. The BODY-Q scales scores are computed from the responses to the items, which are added together and converted to a scale from 0 (worst) to 100 (best). In the final phase, the BODY-Q was further examined for its responsiveness to measuring clinical change.[22,23]

The BODY-Q was field-tested in the United States, Canada, and the United Kingdom.[21] Internationally, the BODY-Q is currently available in 13 languages. These translations followed recommended methodology for the translation, linguistic validation, and cultural adaption process, which ensured that items did not differ in their meaning across different language versions.[31–35] In addition, the Danish team conducted a full psychometric validation study.[36]

BODY-Q Data in Cosmetic Abdominoplasty

To show how the BODY-Q can be used in cosmetic abdominoplasty research or clinical practice, this article presents an example based on data from the field-test study of the BODY-Q. In this multicenter study performed in cosmetic surgery clinics in Hamilton, Vancouver, Mississauga (Canada), and Atlanta (United States), the sample included 234 patients who were before or after body contouring. In the survey, these participants were asked the following questions:

1. What body contouring procedures are you here about today?
2. Have you had the body contouring procedure you are here about today?
   a. Yes, I am a postoperative patient
   b. No, I am a preoperative patient

There were 157 participants who were seeking or had undergone an abdominoplasty. The sample included 111 from the United States and 46 from Canada. Most participants were female (n = 151) and white (n = 111), with the mean age 44 years (standard deviation [SD] = 9.5; range, 20–72 years). The sample was primarily cross-sectional: 140 participants who completed the BODY-Q once (37 preoperative and 103 postoperative) and 17 participants who completed the BODY-Q twice (preoperative and postoperative). The results for these 2 groups are presented separately later.

Table 2 shows the results of the cross-sectional data. The mean score for the scales measuring satisfaction with abdomen and body was lower for the preoperative sample compared with the sample who underwent abdominoplasty. For the HR-QOL scales, participants exploring or seeking abdominoplasty reported significantly lower levels of body image and sexual well-being compared with participants who underwent abdominoplasty. Psychological and social well-being scores were not significantly different between the 2 samples. **Figs. 1** and **2** show the mean scores for the BODY-Q scales by clinical group (before or after body contouring).

Table 3 shows results for the prospectively collected data. Despite the small sample, significant improvement was reported on 5 of the 7 scales (body, abdomen, skin, body image, sexual). Participants did not improve in psychological and social well-being. Participants showed the

Table 2
Mean scores for BODY-Q scales by clinical group (before or after body contouring)

Scale	Clinical Group	N	Mean Score (SD)	P Value
Body	Preoperative	37	41.0 (19.9)	<.001
	Postoperative	103	65.7 (20.7)	—
Abdomen	Preoperative	24	24.0 (24.5)	<.001
	Postoperative	98	75.9 (21.6)	—
Skin	Preoperative	29	33.5 (23.7)	.584
	Postoperative	29	38.7 (28.4)	—
Body image	Preoperative	36	42.9 (21.6)	<.001
	Postoperative	96	67.0 (24.9)	—
Psycho-logical	Preoperative	36	80.3 (18.5)	.872
	Postoperative	96	79.7 (18.3)	—
Social	Preoperative	37	78.2 (19.5)	.834
	Postoperative	96	79.4 (18.0)	—
Sexual	Preoperative	37	58.8 (23.0)	.004
	Postoperative	94	71.2 (22.9)	—

P value is for Mann-Whitney U test.

greatest improvement on the satisfaction with abdomen scale. To understand what the mean scores mean clinically, **Fig. 3** shows the pattern of answers for the sample for the 7 items of the BODY-Q body image scale. Preoperatively, participants' mean score indicated that they somewhat agreed that they feel positive about their bodies and that they like their bodies even though they are not perfect, and somewhat disagreed with the other 5 items on the scale. After surgery, participants' mean score shows that they improved on all items of the scale by 1 or 2 categories.

These data provide insight into how appearance and HR-QOL outcomes differ between patients exploring or seeking abdominoplasty and patients who undergo abdominoplasty. Patients who underwent abdominoplasty were more satisfied with their abdomens and had greater HR-QOL. The knowledge gained from these data can inform

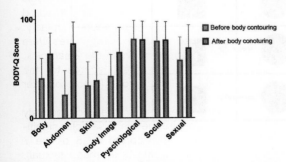

Fig. 1. Mean scores for BODY-Q scale scores by clinical group.

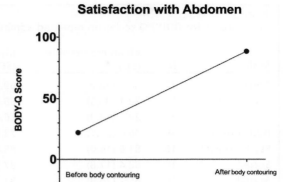

Fig. 2. Mean scores for BODY-Q scales on repeated administration.

patient decision making by understanding the expected appearance and HR-QOL outcomes after cosmetic abdominoplasty. The individual patients can then weigh the expected benefits from a patient's perspective against the risks of these procedures. This example was one that cosmetic surgeons can use in their clinical practice, whereas researchers interested in cosmetic abdominoplasty can use the scales in comparative effectiveness research. For example, researchers can compare different abdominoplasty techniques using the BODY-Q abdomen scale, which may help to decide which procedure is superior from a patient's perspective.

DISCUSSION

Surgeons performing cosmetic abdominoplasty strive for high levels of patient satisfaction and improved quality of life for their patients. Measuring surgical outcomes in an objective and reliable manner will help inform both patients and surgeons of the impact of different types of elective abdominal contouring procedures. Surgical success in cosmetic abdominoplasty is not defined by the absence of complications; it is defined by patient satisfaction and improved HR-QOL.

The BODY-Q is a condition-specific PROM that enables a comprehensive assessment of outcomes that are specific to patients undergoing body contouring procedures such as abdominoplasty. The BODY-Q scales were designed to be responsive to the effects of abdominoplasty on HR-QOL and appearance outcomes. The BODY-Q covers a range of content domains that matter to patients undergoing these procedures, and the independently functioning scales enable surgeons to tailor the BODY-Q to their needs. The inclusion of abdomen-specific items and postoperative items on scarring makes the BODY-Q

Table 3
Mean scores for BODY-Q scales on repeated administration

Scale	N	Mean Preoperative (SD)	Mean Postoperative (SD)	Mean Difference (SD)	P Value
Body	17	38.9 (26.2)	69.8 (19.5)	30.9	.001
Abdomen	12	22.1 (35.5)	88.5 (20.7)	66.4	.003
Skin	7	22.1 (14.3)	56.4 (31.7)	34.3	.028
Body image	16	40.4 (27.1)	73.5 (19.7)	33.1	.001
Psychological	16	81.8 (16.0)	85.0 (19.8)	3.2	.484
Social	16	82.4 (17.8)	87.5 (14.3)	5.1	.123
Sexual	16	65.2 (20.8)	81.1 (25.0)	15.9	.028

P value is for Wilcoxon signed rank test.

useful to measure differences in outcomes between different abdominoplasty techniques.

The BODY-Q also includes a Satisfaction with Care domain, which is composed of scales that evaluate the patient experience with health care.

This domain has different scales that measure satisfaction with surgeon, office staff, medical team, and information. Patient experience is considered a key element of quality in health care. These scales can be used by cosmetic

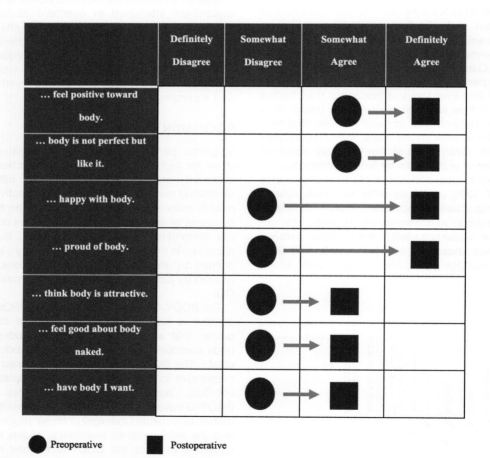

Fig. 3. BODY-Q Body Image scale responses by item and response category for preoperative and postoperative participants.

surgeons to assess the quality of care they provide to patients and offer surgeons insight as to how to improve the delivery of care and patient experience.

A previous study assessed how the implementation of the BODY-Q electronically in outpatient cosmetic surgery clinics was received by patients and cosmetic surgeons.[37] The cosmetic surgeons who participated in the study recognized the importance of routine collection of PROMs in their clinical practice. The routine collection of BODY-Q data could enrich the clinic visits by providing valuable insight into patient concerns.

The BODY-Q is available in multiple languages and the different language versions provide means for outcome data to be collected and compared nationally and internationally. The BODY-Q is already being used in the Royal College of Surgeons in the United Kingdom national quality-improvement initiative for cosmetic surgery service providers. Specifically, the scales relating to satisfaction with abdomen and body are used to collect data from patients undergoing abdominoplasty and liposuction procedures. Data from this initiative will be used to inform decision making and support quality improvement. Further application of the BODY-Q in cosmetic clinics internationally may give rise to better understanding of abdominoplasty outcomes and, thereby, optimize the care delivered to patients undergoing these procedures.

DISCLOSURE

Conflicts of interest: The authors have no competing interests to report.

Disclosure: The BODY-Q is jointly owned by Memorial Sloan-Kettering Cancer Center and McMaster University. Drs Pusic and Klassen are codevelopers of the BODY-Q and, as such, receive a share of any license revenues based on the inventor sharing policies of these 2 institutions.

REFERENCES

1. American Society for Aesthetic Plastic Surgery. Cosmetic surgery national data bank statistics 2018. Available at: https://www.surgery.org/sites/default/files/ASAPS-Stats2018.pdf. Accessed December, 2019.
2. The American Society for Aesthetic Plastic Surgery's cosmetic surgery national data bank: Statistics 2018. Aesthet Surg J 2019;39(Supplement_4):1–27.
3. Matarasso A, Matarasso DM, Matarasso EJ. Abdominoplasty: classic principles and technique. Clin Plast Surg 2014;41(4):655–72.
4. Trussler AP, Kurkjian TJ, Hatef DA, et al. Refinements in abdominoplasty: a critical outcomes analysis over a 20-year period. Plast Reconstr Surg 2010;126(3):1063–74.
5. Boudreault DJ, Sieber DA. Getting the best results in abdominoplasty: current advanced concepts. Plast Reconstr Surg 2019;143(3):628e–36e.
6. Shestak KC, Rios L, Pollock TA, et al. Evidenced-based approach to abdominoplasty update. Aesthet Surg J 2019;39(6):628–42.
7. Rosenfield LK, Davis CR. Evidence-based abdominoplasty review with body contouring algorithm. Aesthet Surg J 2019;39(6):643–61.
8. Staalesen T, Elander A, Strandell A, et al. A systematic review of outcomes of abdominoplasty. J Plast Surg Hand Surg 2012;46(3–4):139–44.
9. Patrick DL, Burke LB, Powers JH, et al. Patient-reported outcomes to support medical product labeling claims: FDA perspective. Value Health 2007;10(Suppl 2):S125–37.
10. Lane SJ, Heddle NM, Arnold E, et al. A review of randomized controlled trials comparing the effectiveness of hand held computers with paper methods for data collection. BMC Med Inform Decis Mak 2006;6:23.
11. Wu AW, Kharrazi H, Boulware LE, et al. Measure once, cut twice–adding patient-reported outcome measures to the electronic health record for comparative effectiveness research. J Clin Epidemiol 2013;66(8 Suppl):S12–20.
12. Basch E, Deal AM, Kris MG, et al. Symptom monitoring with patient-reported outcomes during routine cancer treatment: a randomized controlled trial. J Clin Oncol 2016;34(6):557–65.
13. Boyce MB, Browne JP. Does providing feedback on patient-reported outcomes to healthcare professionals result in better outcomes for patients? A systematic review. Qual Life Res 2013;22(9):2265–78.
14. Kotronoulas G, Kearney N, Maguire R, et al. What is the value of the routine use of patient-reported outcome measures toward improvement of patient outcomes, processes of care, and health service outcomes in cancer care? A systematic review of controlled trials. J Clin Oncol 2014;32(14):1480–501.
15. Bolton MA, Pruzinsky T, Cash TF, et al. Measuring outcomes in plastic surgery: body image and quality of life in abdominoplasty patients. Plast Reconstr Surg 2003;112(2):619–25 [discussion: 626–7].
16. Papadopulos NA, Meier AC, Henrich G, et al. Aesthetic abdominoplasty has a positive impact on quality of life prospectively. J Plast Reconstr Aesthet Surg 2019;72(5):813–20.
17. Papadopulos NA, Staffler V, Mirceva V, et al. Does abdominoplasty have a positive influence on quality of life, self-esteem, and emotional stability? Plast Reconstr Surg 2012;129(6):957e–62e.
18. Saariniemi KM, Salmi AM, Peltoniemi HH, et al. Abdominoplasty improves quality of life, psychological

distress, and eating disorder symptoms: a prospective study. Plast Surg Int 2014;2014:197232.

19. Mokkink LB, Terwee CB, Patrick DL, et al. The COSMIN study reached international consensus on taxonomy, terminology, and definitions of measurement properties for health-related patient-reported outcomes. J Clin Epidemiol 2010;63(7):737–45.

20. de Vries CEE, Kalff MC, Prinsen CAC, et al. Recommendations on the most suitable quality-of-life measurement instruments for bariatric and body contouring surgery: a systematic review. Obes Rev 2018;19(10):1395–411.

21. Klassen AF, Cano SJ, Alderman A, et al. The BODY-Q: a patient-reported outcome instrument for weight loss and body contouring treatments. Plast Reconstr Surg Glob Open 2016;4(4):e679.

22. Klassen AF, Cano SJ, Kaur M, et al. Further psychometric validation of the BODY-Q: ability to detect change following bariatric surgery weight gain and loss. Health Qual Life Outcomes 2017;15(1):227.

23. Klassen AF, Kaur M, Breitkopf T, et al. Using the BODY-Q to understand impact of weight loss, excess skin, and the need for body contouring following bariatric surgery. Plast Reconstr Surg 2018;142(1):77–86.

24. Klassen AF, Cano SJ, Scott A, et al. Assessing outcomes in body contouring. Clin Plast Surg 2014; 41(4):645–54.

25. Klassen AF, Kaur M, Poulsen L, et al. Development of the BODY-Q chest module evaluating outcomes following chest contouring surgery. Plast Reconstr Surg 2018;142(6):1600–8.

26. Poulsen L, Pusic A, Robson S, et al. The BODY-Q stretch marks scale: a development and validation study. Aesthet Surg J 2018;38(9):990–7.

27. Aaronson N, Alonso J, Burnam A, et al. Assessing health status and quality-of-life instruments: attributes and review criteria. Qual Life Res 2002; 11(3):193–205.

28. Lasch KE, Marquis P, Vigneux M, et al. PRO development: rigorous qualitative research as the crucial foundation. Qual Life Res 2010;19(8):1087–96.

29. Patrick DL, Burke LB, Gwaltney CJ, et al. Content validity–establishing and reporting the evidence in newly developed patient-reported outcomes (PRO) instruments for medical product evaluation: ISPOR PRO good research practices task force report: part 1–eliciting concepts for a new PRO instrument. Value Health 2011;14(8):967–77.

30. Mokkink LB, Terwee CB, Patrick DL, et al. The COSMIN checklist for assessing the methodological quality of studies on measurement properties of health status measurement instruments: an international Delphi study. Qual Life Res 2010;19(4): 539–49.

31. Barone M, Cogliandro A, Salzillo R, et al. Translation and cultural Adaptation of the BODY-Q into Italian. Plast Reconstr Surg 2019;144(2):326e.

32. Hermann N, Klassen A, Luketina R, et al. German linguistic validation of the BODY-Q: standardised PRO instrument after bariatric and bodycontouring surgery. Handchir Mikrochir Plast Chir 2019;51(4): 255–61 [in German].

33. Poulsen L, Rose M, Klassen A, et al. Danish translation and linguistic validation of the BODY-Q: a description of the process. Eur J Plast Surg 2017; 40(1):29–38.

34. Rillon P, Chateau F, Klassen A, et al. French translation and linguistic validation of a new patient reported outcome instrument: the BODY-Q: a description of the process. Psychiatr Danub 2019; 31(Suppl 3):406–10.

35. Repo JP, Homsy P, Uimonen MM, et al. Validation of the Finnish version of the BODY-Q patient-reported outcome instrument among patients who underwent abdominoplasty. J Plast Reconstr Aesthet Surg 2019;72(6):933–40.

36. Poulsen L, Klassen A, Rose M, et al. Psychometric validation of the BODY-Q in Danish patients undergoing weight loss and body contouring surgery. Plast Reconstr Surg Glob Open 2017;5(10):e1529.

37. Kaur M, Pusic A, Gibbons C, et al. Implementing electronic patient-reported outcome measures in outpatient cosmetic surgery clinics: an exploratory qualitative study. Aesthet Surg J 2019;39(6):687–95.

Printed and bound by CPI Group (UK) Ltd, Croydon, CR0 4YY

08/05/2025

01864694-0010